MyExerciseMedicine for Cancer

Robert U. Newton, BHMS(Hons), MHMS, PhD, DSc, AEP
FAHMS, FESSA, FACSM, FNSCA

MyExerciseMedicine

Brisbane, Australia

Published by Optimal Kinetics Pty Ltd trading as MyExerciseMedicine

Brisbane, Australia

www.MyExerciseMedicine.com

ISBN: 978-1-7642975-1-6

First Edition 2025

Medical Disclaimer

This book provides general information about exercise, health, cancer, and related topics. It is not intended to replace medical advice, diagnosis, or treatment from qualified health professionals. Every person's medical situation is unique, and exercise should always be tailored to individual circumstances, treatment plans, and medical guidance.

While I describe clinical principles and the evidence behind exercise medicine, this information is offered for educational purposes only. It is not a substitute for personalised medical care. Before beginning any new exercise program, changing your activity levels, or acting on information in this book, consult your oncologist, general practitioner, or accredited exercise professional.

The author and publisher disclaim responsibility for any adverse effects, injury, or outcomes resulting from the use or application of information contained in this book. Although every effort has been made to ensure accuracy, medicine evolves rapidly. The author and publisher make no representations about the completeness, reliability, or currentness of the information presented and assume no liability for any errors or omissions.

Dedication

This book is dedicated to my father, Usher Newton, who gave me the earliest reason to pursue exercise as a medicine for cancer. Watching his rapid decline from prostate cancer, and the consequences of being advised to rest, was a turning point that shaped my career. Dad also instilled in me a lifelong work ethic and led entirely by example. Thanks, mate.

I also dedicate this to my mother, Dorothy Newton, who faced ovarian cancer with courage and resilience. She remained active and socially engaged to the very end—something I believe was supported by the major advances in clinical practice that occurred across the twenty years between my parents' illnesses. Love you, Mum.

To our beautiful daughter Talani—thank you for your patience through every relocation, every late-night meeting, and every hour spent waiting in my office. You have always supported and encouraged me.

To José, who has become part of our family—thank you for the happiness and connection you bring to Talani and to us.

And to my wife Lisa—my unwavering partner in life. None of this work would exist without your love, support, and belief in what I do. I love you.

Preface

For as long as I can remember, I have believed that exercise is essential for health, strength, and a meaningful life. I began my career in exercise science in 1980 and spent the following decades studying how the body responds to exercise—first through a bachelor's degree, then honours, a master's, a PhD, a postdoctoral program, and eventually a Doctor of Science. By the time cancer touched my family, I had already devoted many years to understanding how profoundly exercise shapes human physiology. I understood its power long before I realised how much I would personally rely on it.

When my father was diagnosed with prostate cancer in the 1990s, the standard medical advice was clear: rest, conserve your energy, and avoid exertion. I understood the intention behind this advice, but everything in my scientific training told me it was wrong. After treatment, my father experienced profound weakness and fatigue—the very decline that prolonged rest accelerates. Yet I could not change his path. He trusted his oncologist, as most people naturally would. I was an exercise scientist, not a medical doctor, and my conviction was not enough to challenge the prevailing culture of oncology at the time. Watching him deteriorate faster than the disease alone should have caused left a deep and lasting mark on me.

Two decades later, I watched my mother face ovarian cancer. Her experience unfolded in a different era of oncology—one where exercise was no longer feared but encouraged. She stayed active, maintained her routines, and remained engaged with life. She was supported by clinicians who understood that preserving strength, mobility, and function was not a luxury but a critical part of treatment. She lived with remarkable resilience and dignity until the very end. The contrast between my parents' experiences was profound. It revealed, in the clearest possible way, the cost of outdated advice and the power of doing things differently.

These two journeys—my father's decline and my mother's stability—are the reason I have dedicated my life's work to exercise oncology. They turned scientific interest into personal mission. They taught me that exercise is not just beneficial; it is essential. And they showed how urgently cancer care needed to evolve.

Over the past two decades, the science has caught up. We now know that exercise is safe during and after almost every cancer treatment. We know it reduces side effects, maintains strength, preserves function, improves energy, and protects the heart, bones, muscles, and immune system. Most importantly, high-quality clinical trials now show that structured exercise can improve survival—with effects as strong as, and in some cases stronger than, certain chemotherapy regimens. Exercise helps treatments work better. It stabilises the body during periods of enormous stress. It creates a more cancer-suppressive internal environment. If exercise were a drug, it would be prescribed to every single person with cancer.

And yet many patients are still not offered it.

People are told to "stay active if you can," or worse, to rest until they feel better. These statements may sound harmless, but they deny patients access to one of the most effective treatments available. Exercise is not a lifestyle recommendation. It is not optional or cosmetic. It is medicine—biologically active, clinically powerful, and relevant to every stage of the cancer journey.

I have written thousands of scientific papers, trained and supervised hundreds of researchers and clinicians, delivered thousands of conference presentations, and treated many thousands of patients. But none of that matters if the knowledge does not reach the people who need it most. This book is my attempt to make the science accessible, the strategies practical, and the outcomes achievable for anyone facing cancer.

In the chapters that follow, I explain how exercise interacts with cancer biology, how it supports each major treatment, and how to use it safely and effectively—even in the most complex or advanced stages of disease. You do not need to become an athlete. You do not need to push through symptoms. But you do need to understand the role exercise plays in reshaping the internal environment of the body, protecting the systems cancer disrupts, and restoring what treatment can take away.

My parents did not have access to this knowledge. You do. And that changes everything.

— **Rob Newton**

Contents

CHAPTER 1
Why Exercise Is Medicine for Cancer

Two decades ago, the standard medical advice for people diagnosed with cancer was simple and absolute: **rest**. Patients were told to conserve energy, avoid exertion, reduce physical activity, and protect themselves from fatigue. This guidance came from a place of caution, but it produced the opposite of what patients needed. The misconception was that cancer-related fatigue was the same as the tiredness caused by physical work or exercise. These two types of fatigue are entirely different in both mechanism and required recovery.

Extended **rest** accelerates muscle loss, weakens the immune system, increases inflammation, worsens metabolic instability, and drives profound deconditioning — all of which make cancer fatigue worse. What was once believed to be protective is now known to exacerbate side effects, reduce quality of life, slow recovery, and even shorten survival.

Today, the evidence is overwhelming. Exercise is not only safe for people with cancer; it is one of the most powerful treatments available. We now understand that physical inactivity worsens symptoms, undermines treatment tolerance, and restricts the body's ability to handle the stress of therapy. The shift from "avoid exercise" to "**exercise is essential medicine**" is one of the most significant paradigm changes in modern oncology. It reshapes what every patient, carer, and clinician should expect from cancer care.

For more than forty years, I have worked with thousands of people across every stage of cancer — diagnosis, treatment, survivorship, and advanced disease. I have seen what happens when exercise is used with the same precision, care, and individualization as any clinical therapy. People become stronger when decline seems inevitable. They tolerate chemotherapy and radiation with fewer complications. Their immune system behaves more effectively. Their metabolism stabilizes. Their daily functioning improves rather than deteriorates. And most importantly, their survival improves.

In this chapter, I explain why exercise is now considered a legitimate medical treatment in oncology, how it works, and why it must be integrated into every cancer journey from day one.

Exercise Increases Overall and Cancer-Specific Survival

For years, observational studies have shown that patients who exercise live longer than those who remain inactive. But observational studies can only show associations; they cannot prove causation. Critics argued that perhaps healthier patients were simply more active, and that exercise itself might not be the driver.

That debate is now over.

A major international phase III randomized controlled trial, published in 2025 in one of the world's leading medical journals, provided definitive level-1 evidence. Patients with resected colon cancer who completed a structured exercise program had significantly longer disease-free survival and markedly longer overall survival than those receiving usual care. The relative reduction in recurrence and death approached 30–40% — a magnitude comparable to, and in some cases greater than, established chemotherapy regimens.

Importantly, this survival benefit grew over time and continued to widen through a decade of follow-up. That pattern is exactly what we expect when a therapy influences the underlying biology of cancer, not just symptoms. The evidence is clear: **exercise is not merely associated with improved survival — it contributes to it.**

This finding redefines what patients should expect from supportive care. Exercise is not supplementary. It is a treatment with measurable effects on cancer outcomes.

If Exercise Were a Drug, It Would Be Prescribed to Every Person With Cancer

When a medication demonstrates a survival benefit of this magnitude, it becomes standard care worldwide. It is added to guidelines, taught in medical schools, funded by healthcare systems, and integrated into every treatment plan.

Exercise now has comparable evidence.

If we could distill the biological effects of exercise into a pill, it would immediately be approved, widely prescribed, heavily marketed, and provided to every patient as frontline therapy. Unlike many cancer drugs, exercise benefits nearly every patient, across almost every cancer type, and across almost every treatment modality. It has a highly favorable risk profile, produces broad physiological benefits, and does not carry toxic side effects.

Because exercise cannot be patented or packaged, it has been historically undervalued. But its biological effects are real, powerful, and clinically significant. Every person with cancer deserves access to these benefits.

Exercise Reverses the Harmful Effects of Rest

The outdated "rest and protect yourself" approach created problems we are only now fully appreciating. When activity levels drop for weeks or months, a cascade of adverse biological changes begins:

- rapid muscle loss
- reduced bone density
- declining mitochondrial efficiency
- increased inflammation
- worsening insulin resistance
- weakened immune responsiveness
- higher risk of cardiovascular and metabolic disease
- deteriorating mood, cognition, and sleep

These effects amplify treatment toxicity, making chemotherapy, radiation, and targeted therapy harder to tolerate. They also reduce the body's ability to recover between cycles, often leading to dose reductions, delays, or discontinuation.

Exercise does the opposite. It stabilizes the systems that cancer destabilizes — muscle, bone, blood vessels, mitochondria, metabolism, oxygenation, endocrine function, and immune regulation. It restores what cancer and treatment erode and protects against the downward spiral that prolonged rest accelerates.

The shift from "rest" to "exercise as treatment" is not philosophical. It is biological.

Exercise Creates a Cancer-Suppressive Internal Environment

Cancer grows and adapts within a biological ecosystem — an environment shaped by oxygen levels, inflammation, blood flow, immune activity, hormones, glucose availability, muscle-derived myokines, and metabolic stability. When this environment is unstable — low oxygen, high inflammation, high glucose — cancer cells have more room to mutate into aggressive forms.

Exercise reshapes that environment. It creates internal conditions that are:

- better oxygenated
- less inflamed
- more metabolically stable
- supported by healthier and more effective immune cells
- able to maintain mitochondrial efficiency
- anchored by preserved muscle mass (a key endocrine and immune signaling organ)
- lower in excess insulin and growth-factor signaling
- supported by more normalized tumor vasculature

Cancer cells must live within this environment. Exercise restricts their evolutionary options, reduces opportunities for aggressive mutation, and limits the conditions needed for progression.

I often frame this for patients as *ecological oncology*. Instead of trying to overpower cancer — something biology rarely allows — we aim to contain it by shaping the ecosystem in which it exists. Exercise helps the body negotiate with cancer cells, not through sentiment but through physiology. When the internal environment is stable and well-regulated, cancer's capacity to evolve and spread is limited.

How Exercise Enhances Cancer Treatment

Exercise supports and strengthens every major cancer therapy by improving the biological conditions each treatment relies upon.

Radiation Therapy

Radiation relies on oxygen to create DNA-damaging free radicals. Many tumors contain low-oxygen regions that resist treatment. Exercise increases blood flow and oxygen delivery, reduces hypoxia, and improves the structure and function of tumor blood vessels — all of which enhance radiation effectiveness.

Chemotherapy

Chemotherapy depends on both drug delivery and patient tolerance. Exercise improves both. Increased circulation improves drug penetration into tumors. Meanwhile, enhanced metabolic and immune stability reduces side effects. By preserving muscle, bone, and red blood cells, exercise helps patients complete treatment without delays or dose reductions — one of the strongest predictors of survival.

Immunotherapy

Immunotherapy requires a metabolically healthy and responsive immune system. Exercise acutely mobilizes natural killer cells and cytotoxic T-cells, improves T-cell metabolic fitness, and reduces immune exhaustion. These effects directly strengthen immunotherapy's impact.

Targeted Therapies

Targeted agents often cause fatigue, hypertension, insulin resistance, and muscle loss. Exercise counteracts these toxicities and supports longer-term adherence.

Hormone Therapy

Hormone therapies can rapidly increase fat mass, reduce muscle, weaken bones, and disrupt metabolic health. Exercise protects against all of these effects and preserves long-term wellbeing.

Surgery

A targeted pre-surgery exercise program reduces postoperative complications, improves recovery speed, and shortens hospital stays. After surgery, exercise **rest**ores mobility, prevents blood clots, supports wound healing, and accelerates return to independence.

Exercise is not complementary care. It is a treatment that amplifies the performance of other treatments.

Exercise Improves Treatment Tolerance — Which Improves Survival

Many effective therapies fail not because they are ineffective, but because the patient cannot tolerate them. Fatigue, weakness, nausea, metabolic instability, neuropathy, and deconditioning often lead to cancelled cycles, reduced doses, and unplanned hospitalizations.

- Exercise supports the body through treatment by:
- improving recovery between cycles
- stabilizing energy systems
- reducing nausea and fatigue
- preserving muscle and strength
- improving sleep and mood
- strengthening immune function
- lowering inflammation
- improving appetite and digestion

By maintaining physiological stability, exercise helps patients complete more of their intended therapy — directly influencing survival outcomes.

Recovery and Survivorship: Rebuilding What Cancer Takes

Treatment, effective as it is, takes a significant toll on the body. Many people finish therapy feeling weaker and less capable than expected. Exercise rebuilds what treatment breaks down. It restores strength, balance, metabolic control, bone density, immune resilience, cognitive clarity, and physical confidence.

Survivors who exercise experience lower recurrence rates, better long-term health, fewer complications, and a more complete return to the life they want to live.

Why I Wrote This Book

Most people with cancer never receive a proper exercise prescription. They are given vague advice to "stay active," which is not enough. Precision exercise oncology requires matching exercise to cancer type, treatment stage, symptoms, co-morbidities, and the individual's integrated physiological profile — including hematologic, hormonal, inflammatory, metabolic, and musculoskeletal parameters — alongside personal goals. It requires safe frameworks, correct dosing, symptom-guided progression, and professional supervision where needed.

This book exists to close that gap — to give you the knowledge, confidence, and tools to use exercise as medicine at every stage of your cancer journey.

CHAPTER 2

Creating a Cancer-Suppressive Environment

When someone first hears the words *you have cancer*, the entire landscape of life changes. From that moment, everything divides into before and after. Most attention understandably turns to what the medical team can do—the scans, the surgery, the chemotherapy infusions, the radiation therapy beams, the targeted and immune-based drugs. These are powerful and, for many, lifesaving treatments.

But over my decades in exercise oncology research and clinical practice, I've learned that another critically important dimension exists: the internal environment in which those therapies operate. Every cancer lives within a biological terrain—what scientists call the tumor microenvironment. That terrain is not fixed; it can be reshaped by what we do each day. Exercise, nutrition, recovery, and emotional stability all influence the chemistry, immune function, and structure of the tissues that surround and support every cell, including cancer cells.

My work has shown that exercise is not simply an activity to "stay fit." It is a biological treatment that changes the terrain. When we move with purpose, our bodies release their own medicines—molecular signals that normalize blood flow, train immunity, rebalance hormones, and calm inflammation. We can, quite literally, build an environment that suppresses cancer.

From "Rest Up" to "Move More"

In the early 2000s, when I began formal research in exercise oncology, the standard advice for people with cancer was still rest. The reasoning seemed sound: cancer and its treatments cause exhaustion, so conserving energy must help recovery.

I had seen the flaw in that logic long before. When my father was treated for prostate cancer, he was told to rest until the fatigue passed. Instead, he became progressively weaker, his muscles wasted, and his energy declined even further. Rest did not restore him—it accelerated his deterioration.

When we ask the body to do less, it adapts by reducing capacity. Inactivity produces a downward spiral: loss of muscle and bone, reduced cardiovascular fitness, worsening fatigue, and increased psychological distress.

At the same time, evidence was emerging that patients who exercised during and after treatment not only felt better but lived longer. Early skeptics dismissed this as coincidence—perhaps only healthier people were capable of exercise. Two decades of rigorous trials have since overturned that view. Exercise is safe for most people across virtually all cancer types and treatment phases when it is properly screened and prescribed, and its physiological effects are now well defined. It is not a luxury or an optional hobby; it is therapy.

Muscles—More Than Motors

Most people think of muscles as mechanical engines that move the body. In reality, they are also dynamic endocrine organs—biochemical factories that release signaling molecules into the bloodstream whenever they contract. These molecules, called myokines, are one of the most important discoveries in modern exercise medicine.

When I describe myokines to patients, I often call them the body's internal pharmacy. Dozens have been identified—including interleukin-6 in its beneficial exercise form, SPARC, and irisin—each influencing metabolism, immunity, nutrient handling, and even tumor biology.

In laboratory studies, some myokines act directly on cancer cells, slowing their growth or triggering apoptosis (programed cell death), and emerging human research suggests similar pathways may operate in people. Others mobilize immune cells such as natural killer and cytotoxic T cells—the body's precision weapons against abnormal cells. A further group counters the pro-inflammatory hormones secreted by fat tissue, restoring balance between growth and suppression signals.

Every meaningful muscle contraction, whether from walking briskly, performing squats, or completing an interval on a stationary bike, releases these agents into circulation. In effect, each bout of exercise delivers a carefully dosed infusion of anti-cancer medicine produced within the body itself.

This is the biological foundation of the phrase *exercise is medicine.* The myokine response is tightly coordinated with other systems—endocrine, vascular, immune, and neural—and it works in harmony with conventional therapies rather than against them.

Immunity Retrained

Cancer often develops because it learns to evade the immune system. Under normal conditions, immune cells patrol the body continuously, destroying rogue or damaged cells before they can form tumors. Cancer cells, however, can hide by altering surface markers, secreting deceptive signals, or exhausting the very T cells meant to destroy them.

Exercise can counter several of these processes. During physical activity, the sympathetic nervous system releases adrenaline and noradrenaline. These hormones act as an internal alarm, calling immune cells into active circulation. Natural killer (NK) cells—the rapid-response team of immunity—surge into the bloodstream within minutes of starting to move. Cytotoxic T cells and antigen-presenting cells follow, scanning tissues for abnormal targets.

Repeated regularly, this mobilizing effect can help retrain the immune system. Studies show that the pool of effective NK and memory T cells can expand, while the proportion of senescent, exhausted cells declines. The system becomes more vigilant and better balanced—aggressive toward threats, restrained toward healthy tissue.

I often describe this to patients as a tune-up of immune surveillance. Just as we service a vehicle to maintain performance, each session of exercise "services" immunity, improving response times and coordination. Over weeks and months, the baseline efficiency of the system rises.

In animal and human studies, tumors in regularly exercising subjects contain more activated immune cells and fewer immune-suppressive ones. Exercise helps the immune system see cancer again—and act on it.

Blood Flow and Oxygen—Re-engineering the Tumor

Solid tumors are poorly engineered organs. As they expand, they hijack the body's blood-vessel-building machinery but do so chaotically, creating twisted, leaky, and inefficient networks. The result is patchy perfusion and large regions starved of oxygen—a state called hypoxia.

Hypoxia drives aggressive behavior. Cancer cells adapt by switching to low-oxygen metabolism, which promotes invasion, metastasis, and resistance to therapy. Radiation and many chemotherapeutic agents rely on oxygen to generate the free-radical damage that kills cancer cells; in a hypoxic tumor, their effect is blunted. Immune cells also struggle to function in these hostile, acidic conditions.

Exercise changes aspects of that architecture. Each session raises cardiac output, dilates blood vessels, and increases shear stress on the vascular lining. Repeated exposure stimulates angiogenic and vascular factors that, in animal models, remodel tumor vasculature toward more functional networks. In people, we see improved perfusion and oxygenation that are consistent with this remodeling.

Each exercise session provides an immediate surge in blood flow and oxygen tension—that is, the amount of oxygen available within tissues—and this effect can persist for several hours. When it is safe to do so, I often encourage light-to-moderate aerobic activity shortly before radiation therapy, because the increased oxygenation at that moment may amplify the biological effect of the radiation dose.

With regular training, these transient boosts become structural: capillary density rises, endothelial function improves, and perfusion remains steadier between treatments. This stability matters because chronic oxygen deprivation inside tumors creates evolutionary pressure that favors more aggressive cancer cell clones. By reducing hypoxia and its fluctuations, exercise may lower this pressure and reduce the chances that resistant or metastatic cell populations gain an advantage.

Exercise influences the tumor environment from the inside, making it more accessible to medicine.

The Muscle–Fat Balance

Body composition—the ratio of muscle to fat—matters far more than most people realize. For years, clinical attention focused mainly on excess body fat as a cancer risk factor, and rightly so: excess adipose tissue drives chronic inflammation, alters hormone balance, and disrupts insulin signaling. But more recent evidence shows that muscle mass is an even stronger determinant of how patients respond to therapy and how well they live afterward.

Loss of muscle, or sarcopenia, is one of the most dangerous yet overlooked complications of cancer and its treatments. Sarcopenic patients experience more surgical complications, tolerate chemotherapy poorly, and have shorter survival. Low muscle is not simply a cosmetic or functional issue; it changes physiology in ways that influence disease trajectory.

Muscles are the body's protein reserves, metabolic engines, and endocrine organs that release protective myokines. Every kilogram of muscle represents a pharmacy of anti-cancer molecules and a buffer against the catabolic stress of treatment. When muscle declines, that internal pharmacy shrinks.

This is why I treat resistance training not as optional conditioning but as core medical therapy. Lifting weights, using resistance bands, or performing controlled body-weight movements stimulates muscle protein synthesis, maintains bone density, and preserves functional independence. It also stabilizes blood glucose, reduces inflammation, and restores a sense of physical competence.

I tell patients: every repetition is a prescription. Each time you train a muscle close to its capacity, you're refilling that internal pharmacy and re-establishing the metabolic stability your treatments demand.

Nutrition—Fueling the Terrain

If exercise provides the signal, nutrition provides the substrate. Food determines the quality of the internal terrain on which all these adaptive processes occur.

Over decades of research, the pattern that consistently supports both general and oncologic health is a Mediterranean-style, plant-forward diet: abundant vegetables and fruits, legumes, nuts, seeds, whole grains, olive oil, and modest amounts of fish or poultry. This pattern lowers systemic inflammation, improves metabolic health, and enhances survival across many cancer types.

Protein is critical. I generally recommend a daily intake around 1.2 to 1.6 grams per kilogram of body weight, distributed across meals. This range preserves or restores muscle during treatment, particularly when combined with resistance training. In older or frail patients, or during intense rehabilitation, slightly higher intakes may be warranted if kidney function allows.

Timing matters less than consistency, but combining protein with carbohydrate soon after exercise supports muscle repair and glycogen restoration. In practical terms: a glass of milk, a yogurt with fruit, or a small meal within an hour of training is enough.

Fasting and caloric restriction are promising adjuncts under professional supervision. In laboratory studies, short fasting periods before chemotherapy sensitize cancer cells to treatment while protecting normal tissue. Early human trials in selected patients suggest these approaches may improve treatment tolerance and reduce some side effects, but they are not yet standard care and require medical oversight.

Another key player is the gut microbiome, the vast ecosystem of bacteria, fungi, and viruses living in our digestive tract. A diverse microbiome enhances immune function, regulates inflammation, and improves responses to immunotherapy. Exercise, plant-based diets, and intermittent fasting all enrich microbial diversity. In contrast, ultra-processed foods and chronic stress erode it. I encourage patients to eat for microbial health: plenty of fiber, varied plants, and fermented foods such as yogurt, kefir, kimchi, or miso when medically appropriate.

Nutrition, therefore, is not a separate lifestyle issue; it is terrain therapy. Food choices shape hormone levels, metabolic efficiency, and the same molecular networks that exercise activates. Together they form the metabolic foundation of a cancer-suppressive environment.

Key Mechanisms of Exercise Oncology

These are the core biological reasons why exercise functions as a true medical therapy for cancer. Each mechanism is supported by extensive research and helps explain why exercise improves treatment tolerance, quality of life, and, in many cancers, survival.

1. Muscle as Medicine: Myokines and Anti-Cancer Signalling

Every time a muscle contracts, it releases signalling molecules called myokines. In laboratory studies, many of these slow cancer cell growth, reduce inflammation, and enhance immune activity. In humans, these same pathways support healthier metabolism and improve the body's capacity to respond to treatment.

In simple terms: muscle acts as an internal pharmacy.

2. Immune Surveillance: Mobilising the Body's Defence System

Exercise rapidly increases the number of natural killer (NK) cells and cytotoxic T cells in the bloodstream—the very cells that recognise and destroy abnormal or cancerous cells. With regular training, the immune system becomes more responsive and less exhausted, improving its ability to detect and control disease.

This is one of the strongest reasons exercise supports treatment success.

3. Vascular and Oxygenation Effects: Making Treatments Work Better

Exercise improves blood flow throughout the body, including to tumours. Better perfusion means more oxygen, and oxygen is essential for radiation therapy and many chemotherapies to work at full strength. Improved vascular function also helps immune cells and medications reach tumour tissue more effectively.

Exercise makes the internal environment less protective for cancer and more supportive of treatment.

4. Muscle Preservation: Maintaining the Body's Anti-Cancer Reserve

Muscle is not just for strength—it is a metabolic organ that regulates glucose, supports immunity, and helps buffer the physical stress of treatment. Loss of muscle (sarcopenia) is linked to more complications, poorer tolerance of therapy, and shorter survival. Resistance training preserves this essential tissue and keeps the body resilient.

Every repetition protects your physiological reserve.

5. Metabolic and Hormonal Balance: Reducing Growth Signals and Limiting Tumour Fuel

Exercise lowers insulin, stabilises blood glucose, reduces chronic inflammation, and helps regulate stress hormones. High insulin and persistent inflammation are known drivers of cancer progression. By rebalancing these systems, exercise reduces the growth signals cancer cells use to proliferate.

Importantly, exercise also shifts glucose uptake toward muscle and away from tumour tissue, limiting the fuel available for cancer growth. Together, these changes create a metabolic terrain in which cancer struggles to thrive.

6. Nutrition as Terrain Therapy: Fueling Healing, Not Cancer

A protein-rich, plant-forward diet supports muscle maintenance, regulates inflammation, stabilises metabolism, and strengthens the gut microbiome—all of which influence treatment response and long-term health.

Food shapes the internal terrain. Exercise reinforces it. Both matter.

Taken together, exercise improves treatment delivery, strengthens immune defences, regulates metabolism, protects critical tissue, and produces its own anti-cancer signals—creating an internal environment where cancer is less able to grow and treatments can work at their best.

Stress and the Emotional Terrain

Cancer is first and foremost a biological disease, but the emotional experience of facing it can have real physical effects on the body. Chronic stress is not just uncomfortable; it changes hormones, metabolism, and immune function in ways that make recovery harder. When stress stays high for long periods, cortisol and adrenaline rise and remain elevated. This can increase inflammation, weaken some parts of the immune response, and make the body more resistant to insulin—all of which create conditions that cancer can exploit. This is why supporting emotional well-being is an essential part of creating a healthier internal environment during treatment.

Exercise is one of the most effective stress reducers I have found. Physical activity lowers resting cortisol, improves sleep quality, and helps restore normal hormonal rhythms. It also increases the production of endorphins and endocannabinoids—the brain's natural pain- and anxiety-modulating compounds. The result is measurable calm, not through distraction but through neurochemical recalibration.

I see this transformation daily in patients who begin to exercise again after months or years of inactivity. Their posture changes, their speech quickens, and their faces regain color. Confidence and competence replace fear and fragility. This is not psychological trickery; it is physiology expressed through behavior.

When exercise is combined with structured stress-management techniques—mindfulness, controlled breathing, counseling, or cognitive-behavioral therapy—the results amplify. The nervous system settles, sleep consolidates, and systemic inflammation declines further.

A calmer mind creates a more stable body. And a more stable body is a less hospitable host for cancer.

Working with Conventional Treatments

Some patients and even clinicians worry that exercise might interfere with chemotherapy, radiation therapy, or targeted therapies. The evidence shows the opposite. In many studies, exercise is associated with better treatment tolerance and, in some settings, improved treatment effectiveness.

In radiation therapy this synergy is especially clear. Exercise-related improvements in perfusion and oxygen delivery may heighten the generation of oxygen-based free radicals within tumor cells, increasing their vulnerability while supporting the recovery of normal tissue through better perfusion and antioxidant capacity. Each bout of exercise also triggers a wave of myokines—such as IL-6, SPARC, and irisin—that attract immune cells into the tumor microenvironment, where they help eliminate the damaged cancer cells left by radiation. The combined effect may be a more effective and less toxic therapeutic response.

Improved blood flow increases the delivery of chemotherapy agents and oxygen to tumor sites, making both chemotherapy and radiation more effective. Exercise also increases the metabolic demand of skeletal muscle, drawing glucose away from tumor tissue. This reduced fuel availability can heighten the metabolic stress that cancer cells experience during treatment. A well-trained cardiovascular system clears drugs and metabolic waste more efficiently, reducing nausea and fatigue. Strengthened muscles help patients maintain weight and tolerate higher cumulative doses without interruption.

Immunotherapy, too, may benefit from exercise. By expanding and activating immune cells, regular training supports the very mechanisms on which checkpoint inhibitors depend. Early studies suggest that patients who maintain moderate physical activity during immunotherapy may have better tolerance and, in some reports, better clinical responses.

Exercise also helps protect against treatment-related complications. Neuropathy, bone loss, insulin resistance, and severe fatigue all respond to targeted exercise medicine. The relationship is synergistic, not competitive. I often tell colleagues: exercise does not compete with oncology—it completes it.

For these reasons, I integrate exercise into treatment schedules whenever possible. A short bout of aerobic activity before an infusion, light resistance work on non-treatment days, or brief walks between radiation sessions can all support treatment goals. The specifics vary, but the principle is universal: keep the body active so medicine can work in an optimized physiological environment.

The era of prescribing prolonged rest during therapy is over. International guidelines now recommend regular, tailored exercise as part of standard supportive care wherever it is safe to do so.

Exercise as a Biological Amplifier of Cancer Treatments

When I explain to patients and clinicians why exercise improves the effectiveness of chemotherapy, radiation therapy, and immunotherapy, I describe it as a biological amplifier. Each bout of exercise temporarily shifts the body's internal environment in ways that help these treatments reach their targets more efficiently and with less collateral damage. Over weeks of consistent training, those momentary changes become structural and metabolic upgrades that persist between treatments.

1. Radiation Therapy—Oxygenation and Vascular Effects

Radiation kills cancer cells primarily through oxygen-dependent free-radical damage. The more oxygen present in a tumor at the moment the beam is delivered, the greater the biological effect of the same radiation dose. Exercise increases blood flow, capillary recruitment, and oxygen tension within the tumor microenvironment. Repeated aerobic activity promotes vascular and perfusion changes that, in animal models, normalize disordered tumor vasculature. In people, improved oxygenation and perfusion create conditions that may enhance the impact of radiation therapy. When it is safe, I often schedule light aerobic activity in the hours before a radiation session for this reason.

2. Chemotherapy—Delivery, Distribution, and Recovery

Many chemotherapy agents rely on circulation and diffusion to reach every corner of a tumor. When patients are deconditioned and circulation is sluggish, some regions remain under-dosed. Exercise temporarily boosts cardiac output, plasma flow, and vascular shear stress, helping drugs distribute more uniformly. At the same time, improved muscle and liver metabolism accelerate clearance of toxic by-products, reducing side effects such as nausea and fatigue. Repeated training strengthens antioxidant and DNA-repair systems, meaning healthy cells may recover faster from oxidative stress while cancer cells, already unstable, struggle to repair the damage.

3. Immunotherapy—Re-energizing the Body's Defense System

Immunotherapies work by re-activating T cells and other immune fighters that have become exhausted or unresponsive. Exercise directly supports this mission. Each bout mobilizes billions of NK cells and cytotoxic T cells, guided by adrenaline and myokine signals such as IL-6, IL-7, IL-15, and SPARC released from contracting muscle. Over time, these bouts expand the pool of functional immune cells, improve infiltration into tumors, and reduce immune-suppressive cells that protect cancer. The result is a stronger, more coordinated immune response that may enhance the mechanisms on which checkpoint inhibitors rely.

4. Hormonal and Metabolic Stability—A Shared Pathway

Across all therapies, exercise steadies the hormonal and metabolic terrain. It lowers circulating insulin and IGF-1, dampens cortisol surges, and restores mitochondrial efficiency. This matters because high insulin and stress-hormone levels feed cancer metabolism and blunt immune function. By rebalancing these systems, exercise makes the internal environment less permissive to cancer and more supportive of therapy.

5. The Take-Home Message

Exercise does not compete with medical treatment—it primes the body so primary therapies can work better. A short walk before radiation, light cycling between infusions, or regular strength training through the treatment block are not fitness extras; they are biological interventions that improve oxygen delivery, immune activation, and metabolic control. In the chapter on precision exercise oncology, I explain how we structure and dose this "exercise priming" to fit safely within modern cancer care.

Endocrine and Metabolic Adaptations—Resetting the Internal Chemistry

Beyond blood flow and immunity, exercise reshapes the body's hormonal and metabolic control systems. These adaptations develop quietly over weeks of consistent training, but they are central to why people feel stronger, clearer, and more stable during treatment.

1. Insulin and Glucose Control

Cancer and many cancer therapies drive insulin resistance. Many people diagnosed with cancer already have insulin resistance before treatment begins. When this happens, cells struggle to absorb glucose, blood sugar rises, and excess fuel feeds inflammatory and tumour-promoting pathways. Regular exercise reverses this trend. Every session increases the sensitivity of muscle to insulin, drawing glucose out of the bloodstream without requiring additional insulin release. Over time, fasting glucose and insulin levels fall, stabilizing energy and reducing the growth signals that high insulin sends to cancer cells.

2. Metabolic Competition—Redirecting Fuel Away From Tumours

Very recent research has revealed a powerful new way exercise influences cancer biology: it changes how the body allocates fuel, especially glucose. Exercise not only improves insulin sensitivity—it also shifts the competition for glucose toward healthy tissues such as skeletal muscle and the heart, and away from the tumour.

Cancer cells are hungry for glucose. They use it at high rates to support rapid growth and division. In simple terms, they behave like engines constantly revving. Exercise trains muscles to become highly efficient glucose consumers. With regular training, muscle pulls glucose out of the bloodstream more quickly and burns it cleanly through the mitochondria to produce energy.

In controlled animal studies of breast cancer and melanoma, tumour-bearing mice that exercised voluntarily had much slower tumour growth than sedentary mice. When researchers traced glucose movement, the results were striking: skeletal and heart muscle in exercising animals were taking up and oxidizing far more glucose, while tumours were using far less. The fuel supply had been redirected.

Importantly, this shift persisted even at rest. After the running wheels were removed, glucose uptake and oxidation remained higher in muscle and lower in tumours. Repeated exercise had effectively "reset" the body's default fuel distribution. Muscle became the preferred destination. Tumour tissue became a weaker competitor.

Inside the cancer cells, key growth pathways such as mTOR were dialed down, and genes involved in using amino acids—especially glutamine and the branched-chain amino acids—were less active. This is exactly what we would expect when a tumour faces limited access to the nutrients it prefers: it is forced into a lower-energy, less aggressive state.

A particularly important finding is that this metabolic reallocation occurred even in obese mice, where the internal environment normally favors cancer. Exercise improved whole-body metabolism, increased lean mass, lowered fat mass, and shifted glucose away from tumour tissue. The fitter the mice (as measured by VO_2 peak), the stronger this glucose-competition effect became.

Although these studies were in animals, early human data align with the same pattern: when people exercise before and during treatment, their muscles become more metabolically active and their tumours show changes in genes involved in glucose and amino-acid handling. The exact magnitude of this effect across different cancers is still being explored, but the principle is biologically sound and highly promising.

I often explain it to patients this way: every time you exercise, you train your muscles to claim more of the fuel that cancer cells would prefer to use. You are not just "burning calories"—you are reshaping the body's internal energy competition in your favour. Over time, this becomes a stable pattern: muscle and heart first, tumour last.

This is one more reason I consider exercise a true metabolic therapy. It does not simply lower blood glucose on a lab test; it directs fuel to where it supports health and away from where it supports disease.

3. Cortisol and the Stress Axis

Chronic stress and illness elevate cortisol and adrenaline. In the short term these hormones mobilize energy; in the long term they suppress immunity, thin muscle, disturb sleep, and contribute to anxiety. Exercise acts like a natural recalibration of the stress axis. Moderate training lowers resting cortisol, smooths its daily rhythm, and restores normal responsiveness. Patients often notice they sleep more deeply and wake with steadier energy—signs that their stress-hormone system has returned to a healthier pattern.

4. Sex Hormones and Anabolic Signaling

Resistance training stimulates the body's anabolic signals. It raises testosterone and growth hormone transiently in both men and women and increases the action of local growth factors within muscle and bone. These changes help stimulate protein synthesis and counteract the catabolic effects of many cancer therapies. For men on androgen-deprivation therapy and women on aromatase inhibitors, exercise does not reverse the medical suppression of hormones, but it preserves muscle, bone, and strength within those limits. I explore these issues further in the chapter on exercise with hormone therapies.

5. Mitochondria and Energy Efficiency

At the cellular level, exercise increases both the number and efficiency of mitochondria—the body's energy factories. This means more ATP can be produced from the same amount of oxygen, reducing fatigue and oxidative stress. Better mitochondrial function also improves lipid and glucose metabolism, lowering the inflammatory by-products that promote disease and exhaustion.

6. The System as a Whole

Taken together, these adaptations create a more stable internal environment: glucose is channeled toward muscle instead of tumor, stress hormones settle, and anabolic pathways are preserved. As metabolism becomes more efficient, patients often notice steadier energy and improved recovery between treatments. Biologically, this greater stability makes the body far less hospitable to cancer growth.

Oxidative Stress and Cellular Resilience—Repairing from the Inside Out

Every cell in the body produces reactive oxygen species—small, unstable molecules that are both vital and potentially damaging. In normal amounts, they act as signals that help cells adapt and repair. When they accumulate unchecked, they damage DNA, proteins, and membranes. Cancer and many cancer therapies tilt this balance toward excess oxidative stress, leaving both tumor and normal cells under strain.

Exercise restores control. It triggers a wave of oxidative molecules during each bout, but this is not harmful; it is a controlled rehearsal that teaches the body to defend itself. Repeated exposure stimulates the body's own antioxidant and repair systems, including superoxide dismutase, catalase, glutathione peroxidase, and DNA-repair enzymes. The result is greater balance—enough oxidative activity to stimulate adaptation, but not enough to cause lasting harm.

1. Protecting Normal Cells

Well-trained tissues, particularly skeletal and heart muscle, build stronger antioxidant systems and more efficient waste-clearing pathways. This helps healthy cells recover between chemotherapy or radiation treatments. Patients often notice less fatigue and a quicker bounce-back because their tissues repair themselves more effectively.

2. Targeting Cancer Cells

Cancer cells already live close to the edge of oxidative instability. When exercise raises oxygen levels and enhances antioxidant control in normal tissues, it widens the safety gap: healthy cells are protected, while cancer cells face conditions that challenge their survival. Improved oxygenation also strengthens the effects of radiation and many chemotherapies that rely on oxidative damage to destroy cancer cells.

3. The Adaptive Threshold

This process illustrates a key biological principle: small, repeated doses of stress create strength. Just as lifting weights makes muscles stronger, transient oxidative stress from exercise improves cellular defense systems. This is one reason consistent, moderate training outperforms sporadic high-intensity bursts. Every well-paced exercise session teaches your cells how to clean up, repair, and defend themselves more efficiently. Over time, these adaptations shift the internal chemistry from fragile to resilient.

How Exercise Enhances Cancer Treatment Effectiveness

Mechanism 1: Vascular Normalization and Oxygenation Repeated aerobic activity increases cardiac output, shear stress, and capillary recruitment. Tumor blood vessels show improved perfusion, and in animal models, exercise promotes more functional vascular patterns.

Therapeutic benefit: Better delivery of oxygen, chemotherapy, and radiation; reduced tumor hypoxia; improved sensitivity of cancer cells to treatment.

Mechanism 2: Immune Activation and Myokine Release Contracting muscle releases IL-6, IL-7, IL-15, SPARC, and other myokines that mobilize and activate NK cells and cytotoxic T cells.

Therapeutic benefit: Stronger immune surveillance; better infiltration of immune cells into tumors; support for the mechanisms underlying immunotherapy.

Mechanism 3: Endocrine and Metabolic Rebalancing Exercise lowers insulin and IGF-1, steadies cortisol, and promotes local anabolic signaling in muscle and bone.

Therapeutic benefit: Reduced cancer-promoting growth signals; better metabolic control; preserved lean mass.

Mechanism 4: Oxidative-Stress Adaptation
Each exercise bout creates a controlled oxidative challenge that up-regulates antioxidant enzymes and repair systems.

Therapeutic benefit: Protection of healthy cells; increased sensitivity of tumor cells to chemo- and radiotherapy; reduced fatigue.

Mechanism 5: Psychophysiological Stability

Exercise lowers resting cortisol and adrenaline, improves sleep, and increases endorphins and endocannabinoids.

Therapeutic benefit: Reduced stress burden; improved mood; better immune and metabolic recovery between treatments.

When viewed together—better blood flow and oxygenation, re-energized immunity, hormonal stability, and stronger cellular defenses—a clear pattern emerges. Exercise does not work through one pathway; it reshapes the entire internal environment in which cancer exists and treatment occurs. The body becomes a dynamic partner in therapy rather than a passive recipient.

Pulling It Together—A Living Environment

When I talk about creating a cancer-suppressive environment, I mean something very literal. Every cell in your body exists within a constantly shifting landscape of hormones, immune signals, nutrients, and oxygen. Cancer cells thrive in one type of terrain—sedentary, inflamed, poorly oxygenated, and dominated by stress hormones. They struggle in another—active, well-nourished, oxygen-rich, and physiologically balanced.

You cannot control every variable. Genes and random mutations still play their roles. But you can exert powerful influence over the environment in which those genes operate. Through daily exercise, thoughtful nutrition, and emotional steadiness, you can build a terrain that supports your survival and undermines the cancer's ability to grow or spread.

I often describe this as negotiating with the body rather than waging war on disease. Instead of seeing yourself as a battlefield, see yourself as a living ecosystem that can be guided with care. That shift in perspective changes everything.

Negotiating with Cancer Cells

For most of medical history, cancer treatment has been guided by the metaphor of eradication. We aim to destroy every malignant cell with maximal doses of surgery, chemotherapy, or radiation. This strategy can be lifesaving, but it also triggers evolutionary pressure. When we attack with full force, we eliminate the most vulnerable cancer cells first. The few that survive are more resistant and, freed from competition, can expand. This is basic Darwinian selection occurring inside the body.

An alternative approach is to manage the disease like an evolving ecosystem. The goal is not necessarily complete annihilation, but containment—controlling the environment so that cancer remains stable and suppressed. This idea underpins *adaptive therapy*, where treatment intensity changes over time instead of being delivered continuously at maximum strength. By allowing some treatment-sensitive cells to remain, they compete with and limit resistant cells.

Early clinical trials, particularly in advanced prostate cancer, show that adaptive therapy can delay progression, reduce drug exposure, and preserve quality of life, and may extend survival although this is still being investigated. It is, in essence, a biological negotiation—using the cancer's own competitive dynamics rather than scorched-earth tactics.

I see exercise, nutrition, and psychological support as extensions of this ecological philosophy. These are not soft add-ons; they are levers that reshape the body's terrain to discourage aggressive behavior and support a controlled coexistence with disease.

Negotiation Beyond Drugs

Exercise Medicine

Regular, structured exercise improves blood flow, reduces low-oxygen niches, and enhances immune cell access. It lowers circulating insulin, glucose, and inflammatory cytokines—drivers of malignant growth. Through these changes, exercise may slow disease progression and help systemic treatments work more effectively.

When patients exercise around therapy sessions—a strategy I call *exercise priming*—they are not just improving fitness; they are temporarily shifting physiology at the very moment treatment is delivered. This supports drug distribution, oxygenation, and immune readiness. I describe how to use this approach safely and effectively in the chapter on precision exercise oncology.

Nutrition Therapy

Diet shapes the metabolic fuel supply on which cancer depends. Dietary patterns that reduce excess calories, stabilize glucose and insulin, and lower inflammation deprive tumors of their preferred environment. Adequate protein supports muscle, while plant-based diversity feeds the microbiome that influences immune efficiency.

Nutrition is not about deprivation; it is about precision. Each meal can shift the terrain toward or away from cancer promotion. When food aligns with exercise, their effects multiply.

Psychological Therapy

Chronic stress, anxiety, and depression alter the body's hormonal and immune landscape. Cortisol and adrenaline in constant circulation suppress immunity, promote angiogenesis, and make cells more resistant to death signals. Psychological care—mindfulness, counseling, meaningful social connection—helps reverse these patterns.

Emotional balance is not indulgence; it is physiology. A steady nervous system conserves energy for healing, supports digestion and sleep, and reduces the biochemical noise that cancer can exploit.

Together, these three domains—exercise, nutrition, and psychological health—form a triad of ecological control.

An Ecological Approach

Working together, exercise, nutrition, and psychological therapy create an internal environment that discourages cancer aggression and favors stability. This is not wishful thinking; it is systems biology applied to daily living.

These approaches:

- Improve immune surveillance and tumor recognition
- Normalize blood vessels and oxygen supply
- Reduce chronic inflammation and harmful growth signals
- Stabilize metabolism and energy regulation
- Counteract stress responses that encourage invasion and metastasis

When seen through this ecological lens, the body becomes an integrated system that can be guided with precision rather than overwhelmed by constant assaults. The goal is a stable equilibrium—disease contained, treatments effective, and function preserved. This is not resignation. It is strategic, evidence-based control. By creating a stable internal environment, we reduce the selective pressures that drive resistant cancer phenotypes and sustain the effectiveness of medical treatments over time.

A Shift in Mindset

This philosophy requires a fundamental shift in how we view cancer. Instead of seeing it solely as an invader to eradicate, we can also see it as a biologically dynamic process that can be influenced and stabilized. Many patients live long, productive lives under this model—not cured in the traditional sense, but thriving in equilibrium.

For many patients, adopting this mindset brings relief and renewed agency. The focus shifts from fearing recurrence to mastering the controllable: exercise, nutrition, sleep, stress reduction, and recovery.

Just as in structured exercise programs we emphasize balance, progression, and sustainability, in cancer management we must apply the same principles. The body cannot tolerate endless high-dose stress—whether mechanical, chemical, or emotional. Sustainable health lies in rhythm, not extremes.

When patients embrace this rhythm—exercising most days, eating with purpose, managing stress deliberately—the entire physiology shifts. Inflammatory markers fall, immune function improves, and energy returns. These are not abstract improvements; they are measurable adaptations that influence survival.

Final Word

Exercise will never replace surgery, chemotherapy, or radiation therapy. But it does something no external treatment can: it transforms *you*. It turns your muscles into endocrine organs that secrete protective molecules, your blood vessels into more efficient delivery networks, and your immune system into a sharper patrol force. It stabilizes hormones, clears metabolic waste, and builds resilience from the inside out.

Creating a cancer-suppressive environment is not about perfection or grand gestures. It is about consistency and intent: a brisk walk today, resistance training tomorrow, a nutrient-dense meal instead of processed food, ten minutes of quiet before bed. These small actions accumulate; they remodel your biology.

Most importantly, they return a sense of control. Even amid uncertainty, you can act with purpose, influencing your own physiology in ways that complement modern oncology.

This is what I mean when I say exercise is medicine. It is a physiological intervention that changes blood flow, immune activity, hormone balance, and metabolism in ways that support treatment and recovery. These are measurable biological effects, not metaphors.

CHAPTER 3

Self-Screening for Safe Exercise

Before beginning any structured exercise, it's important to make sure it is safe for you. This screening process is adapted from the ESSA Adult Pre-Exercise Screening System (APSS v2, 2019), combined with additional checks specific to cancer treatment. The aim is simple: to help you start in the right place, at the right level, with the right support.

This is not a test. It is a brief conversation between you, your health, and your readiness to begin exercise training or increase your current levels. Take your time, answer honestly, and use these results to guide your next steps.

Stage 1 – The Essential Health Check

These questions identify symptoms or conditions that may require medical review before you begin new or more vigorous exercise. Please answer YES or NO to each:

- Has your doctor ever told you that you have a heart condition, or have you ever had a stroke?
- Do you experience chest pain, pressure, or discomfort during activity or at rest?
- Do you ever feel faint, dizzy, or lose balance during normal daily activities?
- Do you ever lose consciousness or have unexplained "blackout" episodes?
- Have you had an asthma attack in the past 12 months requiring urgent medical care?
- If you have diabetes, have you had difficulty controlling your blood sugar in the past three months?
- Do you have any other medical condition that may require special consideration for exercise?
- Do you have new, persistent, or worsening bone pain?
- Have you had a recent fracture or are you awaiting assessment of a possible fracture?

- Do you have known bone metastases that have not yet been assessed for safe exercise loading (if they *have* been assessed by your medical team, exercise is still possible with appropriate modifications)?
- Do you have fever, signs of infection, or are you currently neutropenic (very low level of white blood cells)?
- Has your doctor told you that you have significantly low hemoglobin (anemia)?
- Has your platelet count been low enough to increase bleeding risk?
- Do you experience sudden unexplained shortness of breath at rest or with minimal exertion?
- Are you currently taking anticoagulant medication (blood thinners)? Not that exercise is unsafe, but because you may need to avoid falls or contact activities.
- Do you have new, unexplained swelling in a limb that could suggest a blood clot or lymphodema?

If you answered YES to any Stage 1 question, do not begin a new exercise program or increase your current exercise yet. This does not mean you cannot exercise — only that I want to ensure the program is tailored safely. Contact your doctor or a Clinical Exercise Physiologist (CEP) for an assessment.

If you answered NO to all questions, you can move on to Stage 2.

Stage 2 – How Active Are You Right Now?

This table helps you estimate your current weekly activity. It guides how hard you should start and how quickly you can progress.

Intensity	Sessions/Week	Minutes/Week
Light (easy walking, stretching)	____	____
Moderate (brisk walking, cycling, water exercise)	____	____

Vigorous (jogging, fast cycling, gym workouts)	____	____

Weighted Total = (light + moderate minutes) + (2 × vigorous minutes)

Interpreting Your Activity Score

Total Weekly Activity	What This Means	Recommended Action
<150 minutes	Below guidelines	Begin at light–moderate intensity; progress gradually
≥150 minutes	Meeting guidelines	You may progress or diversify safely; consider advice if increasing intensity

Stage 3 – Other Health Considerations

These factors do not necessarily stop you from exercising, but they help determine how to begin and whether supervision is recommended.

Health or Lifestyle Factor	Why It Matters	What to Do
Older age (men over 45, women over 55)	Higher cardiac risk with age	Start light; consider review if new to exercise
Family history of early heart disease before age 55 in men or 65 in women	Inherited risk	Medical review before high intensity
Smoking (current or recent)	Cardiovascular and lung stress	Begin gently; consider cessation support
High blood pressure or medication	Cardiac risk	Ensure BP is controlled before vigorous work

High cholesterol or high blood sugar	Metabolic risk	Discuss with your GP before high intensity
Recent hospitalization	Possible health instability	Seek clearance
Pregnancy or postpartum <12 months	Joint and circulatory changes	Specialist guidance recommended
Musculoskeletal injury or bone pain	Affects safe movement	Tailored exercise required
Neuropathy	Increases fall risk	Balance precautions advised
Lymphedema or lymph node removal	Swelling risk	Begin gradually; monitor response
Severe fatigue	Safety and tolerance	Severe fatigue is very common during treatment. Light activity is safe and often reduces symptoms.
Stoma, PEG tube, port	Exercise modifications needed	Exercise still safe; seek tailored advice
Significant recent weight loss	Possible underlying issues	Medical check-in recommended
Medications affecting HR/BP	Alters exercise response	Seek professional input

How Hard Should Exercise Feel? (RPE Guide)

Effort Level	How It Feels	RPE
Very Light	Slow stroll, can talk easily	1–2
Moderate	Breathing faster, can talk but not sing	3–4

Hard	Deep breathing, conversation difficult	5–6
Very Hard	Only a few words possible	7+

When to Pause or Seek Help Immediately

- Chest pain or pressure
- Unusual shortness of breath or dizziness
- Sudden joint or bone pain
- Palpitations or irregular heartbeat
- Nausea, cold sweats, or confusion

Summary – Your Next Step

Your Situation	Action
NO to Stage 1 and no major risk factors	Start light–moderate activity unless you have been advised otherwise by your doctor.
YES to any Stage 1 or multiple Stage 3 items	Seek CEP or doctor for guidance
Sedentary, fatigued, or uncertain	Begin gently; consider CEP support

Final Words

Exercise is a cornerstone of cancer care. Beginning safely means beginning confidently. This screening process is not designed to exclude you from exercise but to help you understand exactly where to begin. It identifies whether you can start on your own or whether you would benefit from professional guidance first. Current guidelines recommend: *"that people with cancer stay as active as possible and engage in regular exercise during and after treatment, with programs adapted to their abilities, medical status, and symptoms."*

Many people discover that once they complete this process, much of the uncertainty disappears. You gain clarity, direction, and the reassurance that exercise is not only safe for you, but an essential part of your treatment and recovery. Even if you need a medical check or tailored advice before starting, this is not a setback. It is simply part of building a strong foundation.

Once you are ready, you'll be able to engage with the exercise programs in this book knowing they are matched to your current health, your treatments, and your personal goals. You do not need to feel fit to begin. You only need a safe place to start — and you now have that.

When you are ready, a Clinical Exercise Physiologist (or Physiotherapist in some geographies) can help design a personalized program and support you every step of the way. The journey begins with a single, safe step, and this chapter helps you take it.

CHAPTER 4

Principles of Exercise Prescription

Turning exercise into medicine—what to do, why it works, and how to adjust it through your cancer journey.

Exercise becomes medicine when it is prescribed with the same clarity and logic as any other treatment. In this chapter I explain the principles that guide a safe, effective, and adaptable exercise plan for people living with and beyond cancer.

If you have completed the Self-Screening for Safe Exercise in Chapter 2 and there are no issues requiring further investigation or consultation with your health professional, you can begin using the programs in the appendices at any time. If you want information about a specific cancer issue—such as bone loss, lymphedema, fatigue, neuropathy, or treatment side-effects—you can also skip ahead to those chapters. In this chapter I provide you the foundation you need to understand *why* exercise works, *how* to personalise it, and *how* to judge whether a prescription is appropriate for your situation.

Many readers have never trained in a structured way. That is fine. I introduce each concept clearly so you can apply it in practice, either independently or with a clinical exercise physiologist (CEP). You will also be able to recognise good practice when you see it.

Understanding the two principal exercise modes

Exercise medicine relies on two primary modes—**aerobic training** and **resistance training**. They target different systems and produce complementary biological effects.

Aerobic training

Aerobic (cardiorespiratory—sometimes just called "cardio") training uses large muscle groups in a rhythmic, continuous way—walking, cycling, rowing, swimming. The goal is to elevate heart rate and breathing enough to improve the heart, lungs, blood vessels, and the muscle cells' ability to use oxygen efficiently. Aerobic capacity is central to reducing fatigue, improving treatment tolerance, and supporting metabolic health.

Resistance training

Resistance (strength or anabolic) training requires muscles to produce force against a load—weights, bands, machines, or bodyweight. Resistance training protects and rebuilds muscle and bone, improves functional strength, and maintains neuromuscular control. These qualities are essential to tolerate treatment, maintain independence, and preserve quality of life.

The two modes reinforce one another and both are needed for optimal cancer care.

Before we begin: the language of exercise medicine

A few definitions make the rest of this chapter and book easier to navigate. You do not need to memorise them; they simply give structure to how exercise is prescribed. Do not worry if these concepts are not completely clear as we will revisit and explain and provide more detail in later chapters.

Aerobic terms

- **VO_2max**: how fast your body can use oxygen at maximal effort; a strong predictor of health and survival.
- **Maximum heart rate (HRmax)**: roughly 220 – age (or 208 – 0.7×age for more accuracy).
- **Resting heart rate (RHR)**: your heart rate at complete rest.
- **Heart rate reserve (HRR)**: HRmax minus RHR.
- **Karvonen method: Target HR = (HRR × chosen intensity) + RHR.**

You can also set intensity without numbers using RPE (0–10) or the talk test.

Resistance terms

- **One-repetition maximum (1RM)**: heaviest weight you can lift once.
- **Repetition maximum (RM)**: heaviest weight you can lift a given number of times (e.g., 8RM).
- **RIR (repetitions in reserve)**: how many reps remain before failure (you are unable to complete another repetition); for cancer populations, **2–3 RIR** is effective and tolerable.
- **Volume load**: sets × reps × weight.

Periodisation (planned variation over weeks) and autoregulation (adjusting today's session to today's capacity) are addressed later—they are crucial concepts for cancer patients.

How to use the two modes

Aerobic training: what it does and how to apply it

Aerobic training improves:

- heart and lung efficiency
- blood vessel function
- mitochondrial energy production
- fatigue resistance
- treatment tolerance

Effective intensity typically falls within:

- **60–85% HRmax**, or
- **40–70% HRR**, or
- **RPE 3–6**, or
- **talk test:** can talk but not sing.

- **MICT (Moderate-Intensity Continuous Training):** steady, uninterrupted aerobic work at a moderate intensity—typically RPE 3–4 or the "can talk but not sing" zone. MICT is highly effective for building aerobic capacity, reducing fatigue, and supporting treatment tolerance.

- **HIIT (High-Intensity Interval Training):** alternating short bouts of vigorous effort (RPE 6–8, speaking only in brief phrases) with periods of easier recovery. HIIT is time-efficient and, when scaled appropriately, safe and effective for many people with cancer.

Sessions should usually last **≥20 minutes**, but can be accumulated through shorter bouts on low-energy days.

Weekly goal for most people: **75–150 minutes**, adjusted for moderate vs. vigorous intensity. Each minute of vigorous exercise equals two minutes of moderate exercise. For fat loss, **300 minutes** of equivalent moderate aerobic exercise may be needed when appropriate, but the priority during treatment is safety and tolerance.

High-Intensity Interval Training (HIIT)

Entry-level example:

- 30 seconds brisk
- 90 seconds easy
- Repeat 6 times
- Scaled correctly, HIIT is efficient and often well tolerated.

Resistance training: what it does and how to apply it

Resistance training preserves:

- muscle mass
- bone density
- strength and power
- metabolic resilience
- everyday function

Begin with a load you can lift **6–12 times with control**, stopping **2–3 RIR**. **Train each major muscle group two to three times per week,** allowing at least **48 hours** before training the same region again.

Early on, proximity to fatigue drives improvement. Over time, progress is maintained by gradually increasing volume load—more reps, slightly heavier loads, **an extra set of each exercise**, a longer controlled eccentric phase, or additional movements.

How hard and how much: intensity and volume

Aerobic dose

- **Intensity**: HR zone, RPE, or talk test
- **Volume**: minutes per week at each intensity

Resistance dose

- **Intensity**: %1RM, RM, or RIR
- **Volume**: sets × reps × load across the week

These variables allow exercise to be coordinated with treatment cycles and symptoms.

The principles that make exercise work

Overload creates adaptation

Biology improves when challenged appropriately: muscles repair stronger, nerves fire more efficiently, the heart pumps more effectively. The skill is to present enough challenge to stimulate change without exceeding recovery capacity.

Specificity determines the result (SAID principle)

The body adapts to what it repeatedly practices.

Examples:

- Training stepping strength improves stair climbing; unrelated exercises do not transfer well.
- Machine-based strength transfers only partly to free-weight tasks or real-life function.
- Bones respond to **impact and load—swimming will not improve bone density**, whereas step-ups, weighted exercises, and impact training do.

- Isometrics strengthen mainly at the angle trained.
- Eccentric (lowering) work is particularly effective for muscle growth.
- Slow training improves slow-velocity strength; controlled faster efforts preserve power for tasks like rising quickly from a chair.

Progressive overload keeps the signal alive

To continue adapting, progress must be gradual. Examples include:

- one extra repetition
- a 2–5% increase in load
- **an extra set of each exercise**
- **5–10 minutes added to the aerobic session**
- a slightly steeper hill or stronger band

Small increments are safer and more sustainable.

The FITT-VP framework

Every exercise prescription uses the same structure. FITT-VP is the grammar that makes programs clear, comparable, and easy to adjust:

- **Frequency**: how often you perform each mode of exercise across a week—for example, how many aerobic sessions you complete or how many times you train each major muscle group.
- **Intensity**: how hard you work—set by heart rate, RPE, talk test, or load or RIR in resistance training.
- **Time**: how long the session lasts or how long you spend in a specific intensity zone.
- **Type**: the mode of exercise, such as aerobic training, resistance training, HIIT, MICT, or mixed sessions.
- **Volume**: the total amount of work—minutes per week for aerobic training or sets × reps × load for resistance training.

- **Progression**: how the dose increases over time so improvement continues safely.

This framework allows you, and anyone supporting your care, to understand what has been prescribed, how to adjust it, and how to keep it effective during treatment.

Individuality and trainability

People respond differently based on genetics, treatment, comorbidities, sleep, workload, stress, and previous activity. Personalisation is essential.

Diminishing returns

Early gains come quickly. Later, progress slows—not because training stops working, but because the system becomes more refined.

Minimum intensity threshold

Below a certain effort, the body receives no meaningful signal to adapt. Even on difficult weeks, aim to briefly touch a **moderate aerobic intensity** (RPE 4–6) **if safe**, or in resistance training, ensure **sets stay within 12–15 repetitions and no more than 2–3 RIR**, so the work remains effective.

Recovery builds the upgrade

Training is only the stimulus; recovery constructs the improvement. Sleep, nutrition, hydration, and spacing of heavier sessions are part of the prescription. Treatment can slow recovery; when it does, you adjust spacing or reduce peaks accordingly.

Reversal and maintenance

Capacity decreases when overload disappears. Small inputs—short walks, mobility work, one set instead of three—help maintain gains. Maintenance requires much less training than building.

Variation sustains adaptation

Variation prevents stagnation, reduces injury risk, and maintains engagement. Useful variations include:

- changing **exercise selection** for resistance training

- varying **tempo**, such as a 3-second eccentric phase
- alternating **cycling, rowing, stepping, or treadmill** for aerobic training
- alternating **MICT** (steady moderate intensity) **and HIIT**

Variation is deliberate and purposeful.

Cross-transfer

Training one limb can **improve or slow decline** in strength in the opposite limb via neural pathways. This is valuable after surgery or when loading is restricted.

Interference

Heavy concurrent aerobic and strength training can blunt muscle growth, especially during catabolic treatments (e.g., hormonal therapies). Aerobic gains are usually maintained. If muscle preservation is the priority, keep aerobic work moderate and schedule it away from heavy lifts.

Starting level shapes early progress

Lower baseline capacity produces steep early improvements. As progress slows, adjustments to intensity, volume, or variation—not simple repetition—are needed.

Ceilings exist

Genetics, disease burden, and treatment side-effects set practical limits. Very few people reach true genetic ceilings, but treatment ceilings are real. Recognising them helps focus on meaningful outcomes: strength, function, fatigue control, and independence.

The structure of a well-designed session

Warm-up (5–10 minutes)

Gentle rhythmic movement, light rehearsal sets, and targeted mobility.

Conditioning phase

The main work: aerobic training, intervals, resistance training, or a blend, shaped by the FITT-VP framework.

Cool-down

Gradual easing of effort, relaxed breathing, and light stretching.

Periodisation and autoregulation

Periodisation: planning across weeks and months

Periodisation varies mode, intensity and volume so progress continues without accumulating excessive fatigue.

A simple and effective structure for many people with cancer is to rotate **heavy, light, and moderate sessions across the week**, rather than repeating the same demands every session.

Leading up to surgery, you may maintain moderate volume and gradually build intensity. During chemotherapy, you push when symptoms allow and pull back when they peak, aiming for a consistent *overall* dose across the training block. In the days after infusion, we drop the volume and intensity way down and then gradually build toward the next infusion. I explain this in detail in a later chapter.

Autoregulation: adjusting to the day

Begin each session by assessing sleep, fatigue, symptoms, nausea, pain, and medication changes.

- **Green day**: proceed as planned or progress slightly.
- **Amber day**: reduce sets, load, or interval count.
- **Red day**: gentle mobility or rest; seek clinical advice if symptoms justify it.

The goal is not perfection each day, but steady progress across the training block.

Two examples of how a week may look

Lower-energy week

- Aerobic: three 10-minute moderate sessions per day across five days.

- Resistance: two sessions, six exercises, two controlled sets at a 10–12RM load with 2–3 RIR.

Steadier week

- Aerobic: three 20–30-minute moderate sessions plus one interval session (six rounds of 30 s brisk, 90 s easy).
- Resistance: three sessions, six to eight exercises, three sets at an 8–10RM load.

Both achieve similar goals but suit different energy levels.

Tracking and adjusting the prescription

Track aerobic minutes per week at each intensity and resistance volume (sets, reps, load). Record RPE and symptoms. If recovery was good, adjust one variable slightly. If recovery lagged, hold or reduce.

Consistency and measured progression matter more than isolated hard days.

The bottom line

Exercise prescription uses the same logic as any medical therapy: the right dose, delivered at the right time, adjusted to symptoms and treatment demands. Intensity determines how hard you work; volume determines how much; specificity ensures relevance; recovery consolidates improvement; variation sustains progress; and autoregulation and periodisation make exercise workable during cancer treatment.

With these principles, you can understand the rationale behind exercise programs, discuss them confidently with clinicians, and feel more comfortable and informed in any gym or exercise clinic.

CHAPTER 5

Principles of Resistance Training

Resistance training is one of the most powerful tools available to people living with or beyond cancer. The evidence is now overwhelming that it is safe, feasible, and effective across cancer types and treatment phases when prescribed correctly. Major oncology and sports medicine bodies now recommend resistance training as part of standard supportive care.

The benefits are broad. Resistance training:

- Preserves and restores muscle mass, which is often lost during treatment.
- Improves bone health and reduces fracture risk, especially in therapy-induced bone loss or osteoporosis.
- Enhances daily function—standing, climbing stairs, carrying groceries, and maintaining independence.
- Reduces treatment side effects, including fatigue, neuropathy, and lymphedema.
- Improves mood, confidence, and quality of life.
- Supports cardiometabolic health, countering weight gain, insulin resistance, and metabolic syndrome that are common during and after treatment.

For people at risk of cachexia or sarcopenia, resistance training is not just helpful—it is the only intervention that directly stimulates muscle protein synthesis and provides a counter-signal against muscle wasting. Aerobic exercise has many benefits, but without resistance training, muscle loss continues unchecked.

Resistance training is not an optional lifestyle choice. It is a form of medicine, and it must be prescribed, delivered, and progressed with the same care as chemotherapy or radiotherapy.

Understanding Strength

Strength is not a single number. It appears in several related forms:

- **Maximal strength:** the maximum force that can be produced in a single effort (for example, the heaviest weight you can lift once in a given movement).
- **Strength endurance:** the ability to sustain repeated submaximal efforts (for example, how many push-ups you can complete at a given difficulty).
- **Stability strength:** the capacity to maintain posture and joint integrity under load (for example, holding a plank or carrying a suitcase without losing alignment).
- **Power:** the ability to produce force quickly (for example, stepping up into a bus, regaining balance after a trip, or rising from the floor).

All of these qualities matter in daily life and clinical recovery. The same exercise can be biased toward maximal strength, endurance, or power simply by adjusting the load, repetition range, speed of movement, and the rest period between sets.

Muscle Actions, Tempo, and the Stretch–Shortening Cycle

Muscles contract in three main ways:

- **Concentric:** the muscle shortens while producing force (for example, standing up from a squat).
- **Eccentric:** the muscle lengthens while resisting a load (for example, lowering into a squat).
- **Isometric:** the muscle produces force without changing joint angle (for example, holding a squat at the bottom).

Each has specific value:

- Concentric actions are central to lifting and daily functional tasks.
- Eccentric actions can produce higher forces at lower energy cost and are powerful drivers of hypertrophy and strength.
- Isometric training improves joint stability and is used to develop strength at a particular joint angle or within a limited range of motion. This is especially useful when movement is painful or restricted.

Most human movements involve an eccentric phase immediately followed by a concentric phase. This is called the **stretch–shortening cycle**. The prior eccentric action stores elastic energy and activates reflexes that help the subsequent concentric action. Power exercises—such as quick sit-to-stands, step-ups, or medicine-ball throws—deliberately use this cycle.

You can influence which phase you emphasise by changing the **tempo**. A common strength tempo is "2:2": two seconds lowering, two seconds lifting. For hypertrophy you might use a slower eccentric phase (for example, "3:1": three seconds down, one second up). For power, you often use a controlled but quicker concentric phase while keeping the eccentric under control.

Concentric-only versions of exercises can be used when you want to reduce stress on sensitive tissues—for example, using the stronger leg to help lower and both legs to stand up, or stepping up and using a hand support on the way down.

Example. Sally (62) is starting chemotherapy and becomes breathless on stairs. Her sit-to-stand exercise is adjusted to three seconds lowering, a brief pause, then controlled standing. This eccentric-emphasis strategy provides a strong muscular stimulus while keeping cardiovascular strain manageable.

Strength Curves, Resistance Curves, and Equipment Selection

Muscles and joints do not produce force evenly across their range of motion. A biceps curl feels hardest halfway up; a push-up feels hardest near the bottom. This pattern is called the **strength curve**. It reflects the interaction of muscle length (physiological advantage) and joint leverage (mechanical advantage).

The **resistance curve** describes how the external load changes across the range. With free weights, gravity is constant but the lever arm changes. With cables and bands, the direction and magnitude of resistance can shift, sometimes better matching the body's strength curve—sometimes not.

Understanding these curves helps to:

- Match resistance to where the body is strongest and protect it where it is weakest.
- Reduce stress on painful or fragile ranges, especially around joints affected by arthritis, surgery, or radiotherapy.
- Emphasise strength in ranges that are most relevant to daily tasks.

Different tools provide different loading profiles:

- Free weights apply constant gravitational load.
- Cables provide consistent directional tension and adaptable angles.
- Elastic bands increase resistance as they stretch, often matching rising strength through the range.

Example. Priya (42), with shoulder stiffness after radiotherapy, uses a cable row set at a comfortable angle. As her range improves, a stretch band is added to increase end-range load where she feels stronger and less restricted.

Key Programming Variables in Resistance Training

Here I focus on how the main resistance training variables are applied in practice.

- **Repetitions (reps) or time**: a set can be prescribed as a target number of reps (for example, 10 reps) or as a duration (for example, 30 seconds of work). For hypertrophy and strength, rep targets are usually used. For circuit or high-intensity resistance training formats, time-based sets are often used.
- **Load (intensity)**: usually expressed relative to capabilities using repetition maximum (RM), estimated %1RM, RPE, or repetitions in reserve (RIR). In this book I rely mainly on RIR; for most cancer patients, working with 2–3 RIR is tolerable and effective.
- **Repetition range**: for people with cancer, a working range of roughly 6–12 repetitions per set strikes an effective balance

between hypertrophy and strength. Lighter loads that allow far more than 15 reps are usually time-inefficient.

- **Sets**: the number of repetition "blocks" per exercise, typically 2–4 working sets per exercise.
- **Rest period between sets**: shorter rests (<60 seconds) increase fatigue and metabolic stress and stimulate hypertrophy; longer rests (120–180 seconds) support heavier loading and strength or power development.
- **Recovery period between sessions**: a given muscle group generally needs at least 48 hours between resistance training sessions, and sometimes longer in older, frailer, or immunocompromised patients.
- **Exercise type**:
    - single-joint exercises (for example, biceps curl) allow local focus
    - multi-joint or compound exercises (for example, squat, row) recruit more muscle and are more specific to daily tasks
- **Stability and base of support**: widening the stance, lowering the centre of gravity, and keeping the line of gravity within the base improves stability. If stability is a challenge then going to a seated position or using a pole, railing, or wall for support reduces the balance challenge. Progression can involve use of free-weight exercises and narrowing stance.
- **Exercise order**: general principles are:
    - resistance training before aerobic training (other than warm-up)
    - compound exercises before single-joint
    - large muscle groups before small
    - power exercises before basic strength exercises
    - trunk and abdominal work towards the end of the session, to avoid fatiguing postural muscles early.

Together with frequency (how often each muscle group is trained), these variables allow precise adjustment of the resistance training "dose".

Muscle Hypertrophy and Muscle Quality in Cancer

For people with cancer, muscle size and muscle quality are strongly linked to treatment tolerance, complication risk, functional independence, and survival in several cancer types.

Hypertrophy refers to increased muscle fiber size. It is driven by:

- mechanical tension (working near the muscle's force capacity)
- metabolic stress (sustained effort and fatigue within sets)
- adequate recovery and nutrition (especially protein and overall energy)

For hypertrophy in people with cancer:

- Repetition range: about 6–12 reps per set, sometimes up to 15.
- Effort: around RPE 7–8, with 1–2 RIR.
- Weekly volume: typically 8–15 working sets per major muscle group, adjusted for tolerance.
- Frequency: each major muscle group trained two to three times per week.
- Rest between sets: shorter rests (around 60 seconds) can increase metabolic stress, hormonal response and anabolic drive when appropriate.
- Accumulating enough weekly volume without overwhelming recovery
- Coordinating training with adequate protein and energy intake

Muscle quality refers to how much force the muscle can generate relative to its size and how efficiently it contracts. Cancer, inactivity, and some treatments reduce muscle quality by increasing fat within muscle, altering fiber function, and reducing neural drive. Resistance training improves muscle quality even when visible size changes are modest. Patients often report that daily tasks feel easier well before they notice any change in muscle size.

Volume Load and Progressive Overload

Volume load is a simple way to quantify total work:

- Sets × Repetitions × Load.

At the session level:

- Number of Exercises × Sets × Reps × Weight.

Example:

- 5 exercises × 3 sets × 10 reps × 20 kg = 3,000 kg total session volume load.

Hypertrophy and strength improvements occur when volume load is sufficient and increased progressively over time. You can increase volume load by:

- adding a small number of repetitions
- adding a set
- adding a small amount of load
- adding another exercise for the same muscle group

Progression should be systematic and predictable. The "two-for-two" rule is one safe method: if you can complete two extra reps beyond the target on the last set, in two consecutive sessions, increase the load by about 2–5%.

Typical Volume Load Ranges in Cancer Care

For whole-body programs, session-level volume load provides a practical way to scale training to treatment phase, energy levels, and individual tolerance. While exact numbers vary by body size, training history, and the exercises performed, most people with cancer fall naturally into three clinically useful ranges. These are guideposts rather than strict thresholds, and they must be adjusted according to symptoms and recovery.

Low Volume Load (approximately 1,000–3,000 kg per session; 2,000–6,000 kg per week)

This range suits periods when symptoms or treatment limit capacity. It is commonly used:

- Early in chemotherapy or radiation

- During weeks of pronounced fatigue, anemia, or nausea
- In the first weeks after surgery
- When restarting training after a break
- In frail, deconditioned, or older patients

Typical structure:

- 1–2 sets per exercise
- 8–12 repetitions per set
- Light-to-moderate loads
- 2-3 RIR

Purpose:

- Maintain muscle mass as much as possible
- Preserve movement patterns
- Reduce deconditioning
- Support confidence and tolerance during difficult treatment phases

Low volume is not a sign of "under-training"—it is therapeutic during high-toxicity or low-energy periods.

Medium Volume Load (approximately 3,000–7,000 kg per session; 6,000–15,000 kg per week)

This is the **therapeutic sweet spot** for most people with cancer during and after treatment. It provides enough stimulus to build strength and muscle while remaining manageable for the majority of patients.

Suitable for:

- Most individuals undergoing stable treatment
- Survivorship phases
- Hypertrophy and strength goals
- People who have adapted to a basic program

Typical structure:

- 2–4 sets per exercise
- 6–12 repetitions

- Moderate-to-heavy loads
- 2–3 RIR
- Whole body training two to three times per week or possibly 4+ with a split program

Purpose:

- Increase or preserve muscle mass
- Improve strength and function
- Support treatment tolerance and reduce fatigue
- Improve metabolic health

Most patients spend the majority of their training time in this range.

High Volume Load (approximately 7,000–12,000+ kg per session; 15,000–30,000+ kg per week)

High-volume work is appropriate only when recovery capacity is excellent and symptoms are well controlled. It is typically used in:

- Younger or athletic cancer survivors
- Late-stage rehabilitation
- Those with specific goals of significant hypertrophy or performance restoration
- Structured programs supervised by a CEP

Typical structure:

- 3–6 sets per exercise
- 6–12 repetitions, occasionally up to 15
- Moderate-to-heavy loads, often using advanced set structures (cluster sets, supersets, pyramids, accentuated eccentrics)
- 1-2 RIR
- 4+ sessions per week in a split program design

Purpose:

- Maximise hypertrophy
- Build high functional capacity
- Reverse substantial muscle loss
- Restore occupational or athletic performance

High volume is rarely used during active chemotherapy or radiation unless the patient has exceptional tolerance and strong clinical oversight.

Using Volume Load as a Clinical Tool

Volume load is not an end in itself—it is part of the broader prescription. It helps answer two practical questions:

1. **Is today's session appropriately dosed for my treatment phase and energy level?**
2. **Is my weekly training load trending up, stable, or slipping during treatment?**

Volume load also smooths decision-making across changing symptoms—patients may reach their target by doing fewer sets at slightly heavier loads, or more sets at lighter loads, depending on the week.

As a rule of thumb:

- **When symptoms rise**, reduce sets or load to stay within a therapeutic range.
- **When recovery is good**, progress by adding one variable—load, reps, or an additional set of each exercise.
- **Over a full treatment cycle**, the goal is to accumulate a meaningful weekly volume while avoiding excessive fatigue.

Set Structures: Straight Sets, Ascending, Descending, Pyramids, and Supersets

Most patients begin with **straight sets**:

- the same load and repetition target for each set (for example, 3 sets of 10 reps at 20 kg).

As strength and confidence build, more advanced set structures can be used:

- **Ascending sets**: load increases and reps decrease across sets (for example, 12, 10, 8, 6 reps with heavier weights). This is useful for gradually introducing heavier loads.

- **Descending sets (drop sets)**: load decreases and reps increase (for example, 6, 8, 10, 12) to add metabolic stress and time under tension.

- **Pyramid sets**: load increases and then decreases (for example, 10, 8, 6, 8, 10 reps), exposing the muscle to a range of intensities.

- **Supersets**: alternating between two exercises with little or no rest between them, then resting before repeating the pair. Supersets can be structured as:

    - agonist/antagonist pairs (for example, bench press and seated row)

    - upper/lower combinations (for example, squat and shoulder press)

Supersets increase time efficiency and can create a strong training stimulus. They need to be used thoughtfully in patients with fatigue or cardiovascular limitations. These structures are not mandatory, but they are useful tools once a base of technique and tolerance is in place.

Cluster Sets: High-Quality Work with Controlled Fatigue

Cluster sets break a larger set into several "micro-sets" with very short rests in between. This allows:

- better technique
- higher-quality repetitions
- the use of slightly heavier loads, with less breathlessness and fatigue

Example: conventional 12-rep set

- 1 × 12 continuous repetitions, reaching about 2–3 RIR on the final rep.

Cluster version:

- 4 micro-sets of 3 reps
- 10–20 seconds rest between micro-sets
- 2–3 minutes rest between full sets

Total repetitions are the same (12), but form and bar speed are better maintained. In practice I might use schemes such as:

- 2 × (2+2+2+2) with 20–30 seconds between micro-sets and 2 minutes between main sets.

Cluster sets are particularly useful for people experiencing treatment-related fatigue, anemia, or breathlessness. They allow high-quality volume without the deterioration in form that often appears at the end of long straight sets.

Accentuated Eccentric Training

Accentuated eccentric training uses a greater load during the lowering phase than during the lifting phase. This can be achieved with manual spotting or specialised machines that reduce the load for the concentric phase.

Because muscles can produce more force eccentrically than concentrically, accentuated eccentric training:

- delivers a strong hypertrophy and strength stimulus
- is less metabolically and cardiopulmonary demanding than equivalent concentric work
- appears to be particularly effective for fast-twitch fibers and may be less dependent on testosterone pathways

In cancer care, this method is reserved for later phases under close supervision. It is not appropriate for everyone, especially where tendons, joints, or bones are vulnerable.

Light Loads and the Minimum Effective Dose

Light is always relative. For resistance training to stimulate hypertrophy or strength, the load must be high enough that the muscle approaches fatigue within a reasonable repetition range and the load on the muscle fibers is sufficient to produce micro-damage and thus stimulate repair and growth.

If a load allows more than about 15 repetitions with ease, it is usually below the **minimum effective dose** for hypertrophy in someone who can safely lift heavier. Loads below this threshold do not provide a strong growth signal—but they can still be valuable.

Below-MED loads are useful:

- early after surgery
- when pain limits movement
- immediately after a port or PICC insertion
- during weeks of pronounced fatigue or treatment toxicity

In those phases, very light resistance helps maintain joint mobility, movement confidence, and neuromuscular coordination until heavier loading is tolerable.

The key principle is:

- below-MED loads maintain movement and confidence
- hypertrophy and strength require loads that limit sets to no more than 12–15 reps with no more than 2–3 RIR

Severe cancer-related fatigue does not automatically prevent effective strength training. If you can lift a load that brings the muscle close to fatigue with stable symptoms and good technique, that load is usually acceptable. On days when this is not possible, temporary use of below-MED loading keeps the pattern and habit alive.

Lifting to Failure

For any given load, there is a maximum number of repetitions you can perform before you simply cannot complete another rep with good form. That point is called failure.

There is no added benefit for people with cancer (or most clinical populations) in training to failure. Stopping each set 2–3 reps short of failure provides almost the full training benefit with less soreness, less disruption to recovery, and lower risk of form breakdown. This is why I emphasise working with 2–3 RIR rather than "as many reps as possible" sets.

Sessions per Week and Split Programs

A muscle group needs time to recover and adapt after a resistance training session. For most people with cancer, at least 48 hours between hard sessions for the same muscle group is appropriate, and sometimes longer in older, less well or immune-compromised patients.

Practical options:

- Two to three whole-body sessions per week: each session includes all major muscle groups, with at least 48 hours between sessions.
- Split programs: if you train four or more days per week, you must split the body into regions—for example, upper body on two days, lower body on two days. This preserves 48 hours recovery for each region while increasing total weekly volume.

The choice depends on your schedule, treatment plan, and recovery capacity.

What Is a Split Program?

A **split program** divides the body into regions or movement patterns so you train different muscle groups on different days. This allows more total weekly training without overloading any single session and gives each muscle group time to recover.

Common split patterns include:

- **Upper–Lower split**:
    - Day 1: upper body (push and pull)
    - Day 2: lower body (hips and legs)
    - Day 3: rest or aerobic training
    - Day 4: upper body

    - Day 5: lower body

- **Push–Pull–Legs split**:
    - Push (chest, shoulders, triceps)
    - Pull (back, biceps)
    - Legs (glutes, quadriceps, hamstrings)
- **Movement-pattern splits** such as:
    - Day 1: squat and hinge patterns
    - Day 2: push and pull patterns
    - Day 3: accessory or stability work

Split programs are useful when:

- whole-body sessions feel too long or fatiguing
- you want to increase weekly training volume safely
- recovery varies across the week depending on treatment
- certain areas need special attention (for example, legs during ADT-induced sarcopenia, or upper body after surgery)
- a more regular exercise medicine dose is required to address urgent or critical concerns

Split programs still follow the rule that each major muscle group requires **48–72 hours of recovery** before being trained again—split routines simply organise this recovery more systematically.

For many people during cancer treatment, whole-body sessions remain the most efficient format. Splits are most helpful when training four to seven days per week, when tolerance is higher, or in survivorship phases where capacity is improving, or when there is a clinical or compliance need.

Circuit Training and HIRT

Circuit training is a time-efficient method that also challenges the cardiovascular system. A circuit typically consists of 6–10 different exercises performed one after another with short rests, then repeated one to three times. You can also use smaller "mini-circuits" of 2–5 exercises, completed several times before moving on to another circuit.

Circuits can be:

- predominantly resistance-based
- mixed resistance and aerobic
- adjusted to focus on strength, muscular endurance, or metabolic conditioning by manipulating load, duration, and rest.

High-Intensity Resistance Training (HIRT) is a form of circuit training that uses resistance exercises as the primary mode. Typical HIRT features:

- alternating between several resistance exercises (for example, chest press, seated row, leg press, then repeat)
- brief rests between exercises and circuits
- sets prescribed by time (for example, 30–40 seconds work, 20–30 seconds rest) or by repetitions
- rest intervals adjusted to emphasise strength (heavier loads, longer rests between stations) or metabolic/cardiorespiratory stress (lighter loads, shorter rests)

In oncology, HIRT can be very time-efficient and provides both muscular and cardiovascular benefits. It must be scaled to the individual: exercise selection, load, work time, and rest intervals are all adjusted in line with treatment phase, symptoms, and safety considerations.

Another advantage of circuits and HIRT is that I usually implement in a group format which makes it more efficient but also motivating for patients as they are exercising together and supporting each other.

Interference: Balancing Resistance and Aerobic Training

The interference effect describes how high volumes of aerobic training can blunt strength and hypertrophy gains from resistance training, particularly when both are heavy and target the same muscle groups. This was discussed briefly in the last chapter, but I need to give you more detail as incorrect exercise planning can compromise targeted outcomes.

In oncology, interference is most relevant when:

- a patient is sarcopenic or cachectic
- patient is in a catabolic state, for example as a result of hormone therapy
- energy intake is low
- recovery capacity is limited by treatment

In these situations, resistance training is the primary therapeutic stimulus for muscle preservation. Aerobic training remains important for cardiovascular and metabolic health, but its dose and timing must be coordinated.

Strategies:

- prioritise resistance sessions on higher-energy days
- schedule aerobic work on alternate days (preferable) or after key strength sessions, not immediately before
- keep aerobic volumes moderate when the goal is to preserve or increase muscle mass

For patients not in a catabolic state, resistance and aerobic training are complementary and together deliver the best outcomes for function, fatigue, and cardiometabolic health.

Delayed Onset Muscle Soreness (DOMS)

Mild to moderate muscle soreness a day or two after training—DOMS—is a normal response to resistance exercise, especially when a program is new or when volume or intensity increase. It reflects temporary micro-trauma in muscle fibers and the inflammatory signals that accompany repair.

DOMS is more likely when:

- eccentric loading is emphasised
- volume, sets, or load are suddenly increased
- multiple variables are increased at once

To reduce DOMS:

- start with one or two sets per exercise and build gradually
- introduce long eccentric phases only after a base of strength is established
- avoid large simultaneous increases in load, sets, and reps

Gentle movement, heat, hydration, sleep, and adequate protein intake support recovery. Severe or sharp pain, swelling, or symptoms that do not improve should be reviewed, as they are not typical of DOMS.

DOMS is neither required for progress nor a good measure of session quality. Structured, progressive overload is what matters.

Using Concentric-Only or Reduced-Eccentric Training to Limit DOMS

For people who are new to resistance training—or returning after surgery, treatment breaks, or periods of inactivity—the main source of delayed onset muscle soreness (DOMS) is the **eccentric phase** of an exercise as described above. Eccentric contractions place high mechanical stress on muscle fibres, which is excellent for long-term strength and hypertrophy, but can produce significant soreness in the early stages of training as I have explained.

A simple way to reduce DOMS during the first few weeks is to modify exercises so that they emphasise the **concentric** phase (the lifting portion) and minimise the eccentric phase. This approach allows patients to begin resistance training safely and confidently while discomfort is kept to a minimum.

Practical strategies include:

- **Assisted lowering:** Use both arms or legs to lower the weight, but perform the lifting phase with one limb.
- **Supported eccentric control:** Use a handrail, wall, or bench to help reduce the load during the lowering phase of movements like squats, step-downs, or lunges.
- **Concentric-only machines or patterns:** Leg press, rowing machines, or cable stations can be adjusted so the concentric

phase does the work and the eccentric phase is assisted or performed with minimal resistance.

- **Reduced tempo eccentric work:** Instead of a long, slow lowering phase, use a shorter and softer eccentric (for example, one second down rather than three) but this must be controlled to avoid a strong deceleration and stretch at the end of range.
- **Partial-range eccentric loading:** Work through a comfortable range first, adding the full range only once soreness and confidence improve.

The aim is not to avoid eccentric training entirely—it is essential for full strength and hypertrophy—but to **introduce it gradually**. After one to two weeks (2-6 sessions) of concentric-only or reduced-eccentric work, most patients tolerate controlled eccentric loading very well, with far less DOMS.

This strategy is especially valuable for:

- patients beginning chemotherapy or radiotherapy
- those with pronounced fatigue or low training confidence
- individuals prone to severe DOMS
- older or frail adults
- anyone returning after surgery or extended inactivity

By easing into resistance training with reduced eccentric stress, patients establish good technique, build confidence, and maintain adherence—setting the foundation for effective, progressive training in the weeks ahead.

Breathing and Safety

Exhale during the exertion phase of a lift, inhale during the eccentric, and avoid prolonged breath-holding, which can cause marked spikes in blood pressure. This is particularly important for patients with hypertension or cardiac disease.

Ports and PICC lines require specific precautions. After insertion, upper-body loading is paused until the site has healed and you are cleared by your medical team. Once cleared, upper-body resistance exercises are reintroduced gradually.

Example. Jared (43), after port insertion, trains lower-body strength with sit-to-stands and step-ups, while performing only gentle arm movements. Two weeks later, with clearance, he adds light rows and presses, progressing gradually.

Lymphedema

Resistance training does not worsen lymphedema when introduced gradually and progressed sensibly. In many patients, it reduces symptom flare-ups and improves limb function.

Key points:

- start with light-to-moderate loads and progress gradually
- monitor limb sensations and girth during and after sessions
- use well-fitted compression garments if preferred
- avoid sudden, unaccustomed heavy lifting

Lymphedema and exercise are discussed in detail in a later chapter. Here, the key message is that resistance training is part of the solution, not something to avoid.

Bone Health and Metastases

Bone loss is common with endocrine therapies such as aromatase inhibitors and androgen deprivation. Resistance training combined with impact loading is the most effective countermeasure. In the absence of metastases, heel drops, small jumps, hops, and medicine-ball throws can safely stimulate bone, once a strength base is established. I explain this in detail in a later chapter.

For patients with bone metastases, resistance training must be carefully individualised:

- avoid loaded spinal flexion in vertebral disease
- avoid twisting or high torsion through affected long bones
- emphasise supported patterns such as leg press, seated rows, chest press, and wall isometric holds
- avoid impact and uncontrolled loading through the affected bone

Controlled, low-velocity isometric loading that does not create bending, torsion, or impact can be safe in stable lesions when prescribed and supervised by a clinical exercise physiologist. Supervised programs have consistently been shown to be feasible when these precautions are followed. Again, I provide a chapter on this topic later in the book.

Power and Function

Power—the ability to generate force quickly—is critical for independence. Many essential movements are power-dependent:

- rising from a chair
- climbing a step
- catching a stumble
- getting up off the floor or toilet

These movements happen in fractions of a second. When power declines, movements become slower and less certain, increasing fall risk and reducing confidence.

Power training is introduced only once a foundation of strength, control, and safe technique is in place. Strength is the capacity; power is how rapidly you can use it.

Practical power training in this context involves:

- quicker—but still controlled—sit-to-stands
- step-ups with deliberate drive
- medicine-ball passes, wall-ball, ballistic pushups
- box jumps and weight lifting movements such as power clean

The goal is crisp, purposeful movement, not reckless speed. Even small improvements in power can significantly improve stability and confidence in daily life.

Case Examples: Tailoring Resistance Training in Practice

Aisha (48)
Breast cancer, chemotherapy, PICC line, lymphedema risk

Aisha trains three times per week. Early in treatment she focuses on lower-body exercises while her PICC site heals and wears a compression sleeve as advised. Once cleared for upper-body work, she progresses from 12–15 repetitions to 8–12 repetitions at higher loads over 12 weeks. On days with treatment-related fatigue, cluster sets are used to maintain technique and accumulate volume without excessive strain.

Mark (68)
Prostate cancer on androgen deprivation therapy, osteopenia

Mark alternates resistance and aerobic training across the week. He begins the week with lower-body and hip-focused strength work, adds brisk walking midweek, and finishes with medicine-ball passes and balance exercises. He uses the two-for-two rule: if he can perform two extra repetitions for two consecutive sessions, he increases the load by 2–5%. After eight weeks, heel-drop and marching with stamping for impact loading is added for bone health. He notices easier stair climbing and better sleep.

Mei (57)
Stable pelvic and spinal bone metastases

Mei's program avoids spinal flexion and twisting to protect affected vertebrae. Her sessions include limited-range leg press, seated rows, chest press, and wall isometric holds. She works at moderate intensity with longer rests. Over time, her walking tolerance and confidence during transfers improve.

Conclusion

Resistance training is a foundational therapeutic intervention for people living with and beyond cancer. When prescribed and progressed appropriately, it preserves and rebuilds muscle mass, improves muscle quality, protects bone, restores functional capacity, reduces treatment side effects, and supports metabolic and physical resilience.

Meaningful improvements in strength and muscle require training that brings the muscle close to fatigue, uses sufficient weekly volume, and progresses in a structured way. Lighter loads have an important role in early rehabilitation and symptom-limited situations, but sustained progress depends on a clear mechanical and metabolic stimulus.

When resistance training is tailored to your health status, treatment, and goals—and adjusted intelligently over time—it functions as precise, evidence-based medicine. It allows your muscles to actively support your cancer treatment and your life during and after therapy.

CHAPTER 6
Principles of Aerobic Exercise

When we talk about aerobic exercise, we are describing activities that recruit large muscle groups rhythmically and continuously for sustained periods of time. The defining feature is that the energy demand is met primarily by oxygen-dependent metabolism. Walking, brisk walking, jogging, cycling, swimming, rowing, stair climbing, and stepping are all classic examples. On machines this includes treadmills, stationary bikes, ellipticals, cross-trainers, rowers, and steppers. The specific mode is far less important than the system being trained.

Aerobic exercise is limited by the combined capacity of the heart, lungs, and blood vessels to deliver oxygen to the working muscles, and the muscles' ability to extract and use that oxygen efficiently. This is why it is often called "cardiorespiratory training." These are the organs that adapt most directly to aerobic work.

Why aerobic exercise matters in oncology

For people living with and beyond cancer, aerobic exercise is not optional. It is medicine. Cancer and its treatments affect almost every physiological system—cardiovascular, respiratory, metabolic, muscular, hormonal, vascular, and immune. Aerobic training counteracts many of these effects through powerful, system-wide adaptations.

Cardiovascular and vascular adaptations

Aerobic training strengthens the heart muscle, increases stroke volume (the blood pumped per beat), lowers resting heart rate, and reduces blood pressure. Chemotherapy, radiotherapy, targeted therapies, and hormonal therapies all increase long-term cardiovascular risk. Aerobic training directly reduces this risk.

Blood vessels become more elastic, endothelial function improves, and capillary networks expand. These vascular adaptations improve blood flow to healthy tissues and may enhance delivery of oxygen and treatment agents to tumors, where blood supply is often chaotic and inefficient.

Metabolic adaptations

Aerobic training improves glucose uptake, increases insulin sensitivity, and reduces adiposity. These changes matter in oncology because insulin resistance, impaired metabolic flexibility, and central adiposity all worsen prognosis. Improving metabolic health also reduces fatigue and supports more stable energy across the day.

Muscle-level adaptations

Repeated aerobic work increases the number and size of mitochondria—the cell's energy-producing structures—and enhances oxidative enzyme activity. Capillary density increases, improving oxygen and nutrient delivery. These adaptations help muscles function with less strain during everyday tasks.

Chemotherapy, radiation, inactivity, and systemic inflammation all damage mitochondria, reduce capillary density, and impair muscular energy production. Aerobic training reverses many of these deficits, restoring metabolic efficiency.

Respiratory adaptations

The lungs become more efficient at moving air, and respiratory muscles strengthen. For patients who have undergone thoracic surgery or chest radiotherapy, where respiratory reserve may be reduced, this adaptation is especially valuable.

Immune and inflammatory effects

Each bout of aerobic exercise mobilizes immune cells—natural killer cells, cytotoxic T-cells, and dendritic cells—into circulation. Over time, chronic inflammation decreases, immune regulation improves, and immune surveillance sharpens. These shifts support overall recovery and may contribute to improved cancer outcomes.

The power of vigorous aerobic work

While all aerobic exercise is beneficial, vigorous-intensity training—when medically appropriate—produces more substantial adaptations in the cardiovascular, metabolic, muscular, and hormonal systems most relevant to cancer progression and survivorship.

What happens during a session: acute responses

When you begin an aerobic session, your body responds immediately:

- **Heart rate rises** to deliver more oxygen.
- **Stroke volume increases**, and cardiac output can rise four- to six-fold.
- **Blood vessels supplying muscle dilate**; vessels to non-essential organs constrict.
- **VO_2 (oxygen uptake) increases** as working muscles extract more oxygen from the blood.
- **Breathing becomes deeper and faster**, matching ventilation to metabolic demand.
- **Adrenaline and other hormones rise**, mobilizing glucose and fat for fuel.
- **Body temperature increases**, and sweating helps maintain safe operating temperatures.

To the patient, these responses feel like: a faster pulse, warm skin, light sweating, and deeper but controlled breathing. These sensations indicate that the therapeutic processes are underway—not that something is wrong.

How the body remodels: chronic adaptations

With consistent aerobic training, these acute responses generate long-term adaptations:

- The left ventricle enlarges and strengthens.
- Resting and submaximal heart rates fall.
- Blood pressure declines as arteries become more elastic.
- Blood volume increases, improving oxygen carriage.
- Capillaries proliferate in muscle.
- Mitochondria multiply and enlarge; oxidative enzymes increase.
- Muscles become more efficient at sparing glycogen and using fat for fuel.

- Respiratory function improves, including respiratory muscle strength.
- Red blood cell mass may increase.
- Immune function becomes more regulated, with lower chronic inflammation.

These adaptations together raise **VO_2max**, one of the strongest predictors of surgical risk, chemotherapy tolerance, treatment toxicity, recurrence, and survival.

Patient vignette: *Anna's walk*

Anna, 52, completed chemotherapy for breast cancer six weeks earlier. She described herself as "wiped out." We began with walking at RPE 3–4 for 12 minutes. Each week we added two minutes. After four weeks she could walk briskly for 20 minutes, her resting heart rate dropped from 84 to 72, and her fatigue improved. What she felt as "less puffed" reflected real cardiovascular and muscular remodeling.

Prescribing intensity: making it personal

In Chapter 4 I introduced the terminology for aerobic intensity (HRmax, HRR, RPE, talk test). Here I apply these tools specifically to aerobic training.

Using heart rate reserve (HRR) to set zones

To personalise training, HRR is often the most accurate method because it accounts for both maximum and resting heart rate.

Example

A 65-year-old woman with RHR = 70 bpm (measured by smartwatch or pulse).

HRmax $\approx 208 - (0.7 \times 65) = 162$ bpm.

HRR $= 162 - 70 = 92$ bpm.

Moderate intensity (40–60% HRR):

- 40%: $(0.40 \times 92) + 70 =$ **107 bpm**
- 60%: $(0.60 \times 92) + 70 =$ **125 bpm**

Moderate training range ≈ **107–125 bpm.**

Vigorous intensity (70–85% HRR):

- 70%: (0.70 × 92) + 70 = **134 bpm**
- 85%: (0.85 × 92) + 70 = **148 bpm**

Vigorous training range ≈ **134–148 bpm.**

These calculations are intentionally straightforward so that patients can determine their own training zones.

Other intensity tools

- **RPE (0–10 scale):**
  Moderate = 4–6,
  Vigorous = 7–8.
- **Talk test:**
  Moderate = can talk but not sing;
  Vigorous = can talk in short phrases only.
- **METs:**
  1 MET = resting oxygen use.
  Brisk walking ≈ 4 METs; jogging ≈ 8 METs.

Patients do not need to master all methods—using one consistently is enough.

Training formats

Moderate-Intensity Continuous Training (MICT)

Steady-state work at moderate intensity, usually 20–40 minutes. It sits below the *anaerobic threshold* and is sustainable. MICT is foundational and appropriate for nearly all patients.

Interval Training

Alternating periods of harder work with easier recovery. Interval structure modifies the training effect and can target different energy systems. The recovery interval can be rest e.g. standing or sitting but usually best to keep moving but at low intensity (i.e. RPE 2-3).

High-Intensity Interval Training (HIIT)

HIIT alternates vigorous work with recovery. When scaled properly, it is safe and effective in people with cancer. HIIT may drive stronger adaptations in cardiovascular, metabolic, and muscular systems.

There are three main interval categories with work:rest ratios that emphasize different energy systems:

- **ATP-CP system:** short bursts (10 sec) with long recovery (1:3+).
- **Lactate system:** 30–60 sec work with 1–2 min recovery (1:2).
- **Aerobic system:** 2–4 min work with equal recovery (1:1).

Not all patients will use these exact structures, but they illustrate how intervals target different systems. When you work with your exercise professional they may use these terms and prescriptions.

Guidelines and their limits

The American College of Sports Medicine (ACSM) recommends ≥150 minutes of moderate or 75 minutes of vigorous aerobic activity per week (≈600 MET-minutes), but these guidelines are based on relatively healthy survivors.

For patients in active treatment, these thresholds may be unrealistic. The goal is not rigid adherence but **progressive accumulation**, scaled to treatment and symptoms. For some, 10 minutes of walking may be the therapeutic starting point.

Generic guidelines do not account for anemia, neuropathy, bone metastases, or chemotherapy-related fatigue. Precision exercise oncology (see later chapter) adapts the dose, timing, and delivery to each patient.

Patient vignette: *James on ADT*

James, 68, on androgen deprivation therapy, gained six kilograms and developed impaired glucose control. We started recumbent cycling at RPE 4–5 for 20 minutes, three times per week. Over 12 weeks he progressed to 30 minutes with short intervals. Waist circumference dropped, glucose normalised, and his energy improved.

When to Modify or Pause Aerobic Exercise: Safety Thresholds

In Chapter 2 I outlined the general safety screen for all exercise. Aerobic exercise adds its own considerations because it places demand on the heart, lungs, and circulatory system. These thresholds help you decide when to reduce the dose, change the mode, or temporarily pause until it is safe to resume. They are guides, not rigid rules, and must be interpreted in the context of your overall symptoms and treatment plan.

Blood counts

Certain pathology values indicate when the body's capacity for aerobic work is reduced:

- **Hemoglobin <80 g/L:** Limit activity to gentle walking or mobility. Low hemoglobin reduces oxygen-carrying capacity and increases breathlessness, so vigorous or moderate aerobic training is unsafe.
- **Platelets <20 × 10^9/L:** Avoid resistance training and any aerobic work that risks loss of balance or falls.
- **Platelets <50 × 10^9/L:** Avoid vigorous aerobic training and impact-based modes such as jogging, stepping, or stair repeats. Low-impact, steady walking is usually safe if symptoms are stable.
- **Severe neutropenia:** Avoid public gyms and pools because of infection risk. Home-based walking, cycling, or stepping is safe and encouraged unless you have fever or systemic symptoms.

Symptoms that require immediate adjustment

Regardless of pathology values, exercise should stop and be reassessed if you experience:

- chest pain or new chest tightness
- unexplained breathlessness that exceeds your usual pattern

- dizziness, faintness, or palpitations
- fever, chills, or signs of acute infection
- unusual bleeding or bruising
- pain acting differently from your expected treatment-related pattern

Today's plan must always align with today's symptoms. On high-fatigue or high-toxicity days, shifting to low-intensity mobility or short bouts of slow walking is often the safest option.

Medication considerations

Some medications blunt or modify heart rate responses, meaning heart-rate zones are not reliable indicators of aerobic intensity. This includes:

- beta-blockers
- some calcium-channel blockers
- certain targeted therapies
- anti-arrhythmic medications

If you are taking any of these, guide intensity using **RPE** (effort 4–6 for moderate, 7–8 for vigorous) or the **talk test**, rather than heart rate.

Practical decision-making

A simple way to integrate these thresholds is:

- **Green light** — blood counts stable, symptoms controlled → Proceed with your planned session and adjust based on how you feel.
- **Amber light** — low energy, mild nausea, transient dizziness, mild breathlessness → Reduce duration and intensity; consider breaking sessions into shorter blocks.
- **Red light** — fever, chest symptoms, severe anemia, very low platelets, sudden or unexplained breathlessness → Pause structured training and seek medical advice.

These thresholds do not limit your ability to be active—they help ensure that aerobic training remains safe, therapeutic, and aligned with your physiological capacity at each stage of treatment.

Aerobic equipment in cancer care

Aerobic training can be delivered safely using a wide range of equipment:

- **Treadmills:** controlled speed/grade; caution with neuropathy.
- **Stationary cycles:** highly versatile and safe for balance or bone fragility concerns.
- **Recumbent cycles:** supportive and often best for frail or symptomatic patients.
- **Ellipticals/cross-trainers:** whole-body, low-impact, but require coordination.
- **Rowers:** potent cardiovascular stimulus but can strain the back.
- **Steppers/stair climbers:** mimic stair climbing; useful but knee-loading varies.
- **Arm-crank ergometers:** excellent when lower limbs cannot be loaded.
- **Step benches:** simple, measurable, and ideal for home programs.

Patient vignette: *Susan's arm cycle*

Susan, 59, had pelvic bone metastases and neuropathy. Arm-crank cycling allowed her to train safely. She progressed from 5 to 20 minutes, reporting improved fatigue and confidence.

Modern systems and wearables

Modern ergometers and wearables provide heart-rate, cadence, power, and time-in-zone metrics that enable precise, remote-supported exercise oncology. Apps and platforms allow structured intervals, session tracking, and data review (e.g., FitMed www.fitmed.com).

These numbers guide, but do not dictate; symptom awareness still matters most.

Bringing it all together

Aerobic exercise is not background "cardio." It is core medical therapy in oncology. Understanding how the body responds, adapts, and remodels helps patients appreciate why the effort matters and how to train safely.

Generic guidelines offer a useful benchmark but are not the goal. The goal is **personalised progression**—right dose, right timing, right context.

Whether performed on a treadmill in a clinic, a recumbent cycle at home, an arm-crank ergometer in rehabilitation, or a step bench in a living room, aerobic exercise alters the trajectory of cancer survivorship. It reduces treatment side-effects, improves tolerance of therapy, enhances metabolic and cardiovascular health, boosts immunity, preserves function, and restores confidence.

It is not optional. It is essential.

CHAPTER 7
Which Exercise is Best?

"The best exercise is the one that you will do consistently and for the long-term."

Move Every Day: The First Principle of Exercise Medicine

For anyone diagnosed with cancer, one of the most important commitments you can make is to avoid prolonged sedentary time. Sitting still for long periods is a physiological stressor. Even small amounts of exercise provide measurable benefit, but consistency is the strongest predictor of improved function, symptom control, treatment tolerance, and survival. Daily exercise—performed most days of the week, sustained over months and years—is the foundation of exercise medicine.

This is why I often say that the best exercise is the one you will do regularly. If you enjoy cycling, cycle. If resistance exercise appeals to you, make it part of your routine. If dancing is something you find engaging, then dance. The clinical benefit comes from regularity and sufficient intensity, not from the setting or equipment.

Why Sitting Is Harmful

Sedentary behavior is an independent risk factor for poor health, even in people who meet weekly exercise guidelines. Long uninterrupted periods of sitting reduce muscle activation, limit blood flow, impair glucose uptake, worsen insulin resistance, and suppress the release of myokines—molecules released by muscle that support immune function, metabolic health, and tumor control.

For people with cancer, this loss of muscle-derived protective signaling is particularly concerning. Muscle contractions release myokines that influence inflammation, immune surveillance, and cellular stability. Long sedentary periods remove this protective input and allow physiological decline to accelerate.

Breaking up sitting time is therefore as important as structured exercise. Standing, stretching, or performing light exercise every 30–60 minutes helps reactivate muscle tissue, improve circulation, and support metabolic balance.

Everyday Opportunities: More Than Walking

When people think of exercise, they often picture long walks or gym sessions. In reality, resistance exercise can be integrated into daily life. Bodyweight exercises such as squats, sit-to-stands, wall push-ups, and step-ups require no equipment and can be performed in short bouts throughout the day.

Practical examples include:

- ten squats in the morning
- ten wall push-ups before lunch
- ten sit-to-stands before dinner

Accumulated across a week, these simple routines create meaningful resistance training stimulus.

Daily life also provides natural opportunities for loading muscle and bone: carrying groceries upstairs, gardening, lifting household items, or playing physically with grandchildren. These tasks produce real physiological benefit—they stimulate muscle fibers, load the skeleton, and activate hormonal and immune pathways important for maintaining independence and resilience.

Consistency and Enjoyment

Exercise adherence improves when activities are enjoyable or at least acceptable and convenient. Choosing exercise that fits your interests and environment builds sustainability. Social participation also supports adherence; exercising with another person, joining a class, or pairing exercise with enjoyable audio content improves long-term consistency.

Habit formation science shows that linking exercise to existing daily behaviors increases follow-through. Short bouts of exercise after boiling the kettle or before an evening television program are effective ways to anchor routine.

Clinical Examples

These examples illustrate how modest, consistent exercise can be integrated into different lifestyles:

A 72-year-old woman recovering from breast cancer began with a single daily set of sit-to-stands. Over several weeks she progressed to two sets and then three, eventually performing 30 repetitions per day with ease. Her lower-body strength and balance improved markedly.

A 59-year-old man following colon cancer surgery maintained his golf routine rather than stopping it. By increasing the frequency of nine-hole rounds each week, he rebuilt stamina and leg strength, regaining confidence in his physical capacity.

A 44-year-old woman undergoing chemotherapy used her enjoyment of music to establish regular activity. Gentle dancing in her living room for 15–20 minutes most evenings helped maintain energy, mood, and appetite during treatment.

These are not dramatic training programs. They are examples of consistent, sustainable exercise that targets key physiological systems.

Dose–Response: Some Is Good, More Is Better

Exercise follows a dose–response relationship. Small increases from a low baseline produce large health gains. Greater benefits occur with higher volumes and intensities—up to a point—particularly when performed for at least 20 minutes on most days.

Progression must be individualized. For some, this begins with a few minutes of exercise dispersed across the day; for others, structured 20–30 minute sessions are feasible immediately. The principle is gradual progression toward reliable daily exercise.

Is Any Exercise Good Enough?

Any exercise is better than none, but not all exercise provides the same clinical benefit. Exercise should be prescribed with the same precision given to medical treatments.

Different exercise types produce different adaptations:

- **Resistance training** is essential for preserving or rebuilding muscle and counteracting sarcopenia and cachexia.
- **Impact training** helps protect against treatment-related bone loss.
- **Aerobic exercise** improves cardiovascular health, reduces fatigue, and regulates metabolic function.
- **Mobility and balance exercises** reduce falls risk and maintain independence.

Daily general activity forms the base, but optimal outcomes are achieved when exercise type, intensity, and volume are tailored to the person's treatment, physiology, and goals.

The Medical Analogy

Exercise medicine is similar to radiotherapy or chemotherapy: the right type, dose, and schedule matter. No oncologist prescribes "some radiation, whenever you feel like it." Instead, treatment is matched precisely to tumor type, stage, and individual characteristics.

Exercise is no different. The foundation is daily activity; the refinement is precision. When type and dosage match clinical need, exercise becomes a targeted therapy.

Transition to Precision Exercise

This chapter emphasizes the baseline: avoiding prolonged sitting and exercising daily. In the coming chapters, I explain how to progress from general activity to precision exercise oncology—where exercise type, intensity, and timing are calibrated to your cancer, treatment plan, symptoms, and health status.

Key Message

Do not wait for the perfect program. Begin now. Exercise every day. Break up sitting time. Walk, cycle, dance, lift, squat, push, and pull. Build exercise into daily routines. Consistency is the foundation on which precision exercise medicine is built.

CHAPTER 8

What Time of Day Should I Exercise?

I'm often asked, "What's the best time of day to exercise?"

My answer is simple: the best time of day to train is the time that you will actually exercise.

When it comes to dosing yourself with exercise medicine, the key is consistency. I've said it several times throughout this book—small, regular doses of exercise are far more effective than occasional large ones.

It's much better to provide micro-doses of exercise throughout the week than to say, "I don't have time during the week, so I'll just do three hours on Saturday."

Yes, a single big session is better than nothing—but it's clearly not optimal. Think of it this way: if you had a headache, you wouldn't take the whole bottle of Panadol on Saturday and then nothing for the rest of the week. You'd end up in the emergency department!

Exercise works in a similar way. It's medicine, and medicine works best when taken regularly in the right dose.

The Ideal Exercise Dose

As we've discussed throughout this book, the ideal minimum dose of exercise medicine is around 20 minutes per session. If you're experiencing considerable fatigue, pain, or treatment-related side effects that make longer sessions difficult, even five to ten minutes can still act as a powerful "micro-dose."

Short, consistent sessions stimulate the same healing systems—immune, hormonal, muscular, and metabolic—that drive the anti-cancer benefits of exercise.

In general, a daily duration of 20–45 minutes is excellent, with 60 minutes being the upper end for most people.

So the real question becomes: When should you take that dose?

Morning, Midday, or Evening?

The honest answer: whenever it suits you best.

Personally, by the end of the day, I'm tired. After working, teaching, meetings, and everything else, I don't particularly feel like exercising in the late afternoon or evening. So, for me, the best time to train is first thing in the morning.

I'm what's called a lark—a morning person. You might have heard that people tend to fall into two general types: larks and owls.

Larks wake early, feel alert and energetic in the morning, and prefer to get things done before midday. Owls tend to wake and function better later, with more energy in the evening.

I definitely fall into the first category. My wife and I usually wake around 5 a.m., have a coffee, and then start training by about 6 a.m. Our exercise medicine dose is complete by 7:30 or 8 a.m.—and the rest of the day is ours.

That works beautifully for us, but it doesn't suit everyone.

Midday and Afternoon Options

If you're working, lunchtime can be an excellent opportunity for exercise. A 30-minute session fits nicely between meetings, and afterward you still have time for a quick meal and a short rest.

Many people find that exercising during the middle of the day improves their alertness and productivity for the afternoon and helps avoid that mid-afternoon energy slump.

For others, after work or in the evening is ideal. It's a way to unwind, clear the mind, and transition from work to personal time.

Some people find evening exercise interferes with sleep, especially if it's very high intensity. Others—like me—find it actually improves sleep, even when done an hour or two before bedtime.

Everyone's physiology and routine are different. The best approach is to experiment and observe how your body responds.

What Does the Science Say?

Research comparing morning versus evening exercise shows only small differences. Some studies suggest that morning training may help regulate metabolism and improve adherence, while evening training might slightly enhance strength and performance because body temperature and muscle function are often at their best later in the day.

But the evidence isn't strong enough to declare a clear winner. What matters most is not when you exercise—it's that you do it, consistently.

Regularity drives adaptation. Your body thrives on rhythm and routine.

Micro-Workouts and Breaking Up the Day

If work, family, fatigue, or treatment side effects make it difficult to set aside 45–60 minutes in one block, there's absolutely no harm in breaking your exercise dosage into smaller sessions across the day.

For example: 10–20 minutes in the morning, another 10–20 minutes at lunch, and a short session in the evening.

You'll still achieve your total daily dose.

Now, some scientists will point out—correctly—that shorter, spread-out sessions don't create the same homeostatic disturbance as one continuous workout. Your body temperature doesn't rise as much, blood glucose doesn't drop as sharply, and hormonal responses are less pronounced.

That's true. But again, consistency beats intensity when it comes to long-term benefit.

It's far better to complete smaller bouts regularly than to plan one long session that never happens.

The Take-Home Message

In the end, the best time to exercise is the time that allows you to be consistent—whatever fits your energy levels, your cancer treatment schedule, and your life.

Whether it's early morning, during lunch, or after work, the goal is the same: to take your daily dose of exercise medicine most—if not every—day of the week.

Because just like any powerful medicine, it only works if you take it.

CHAPTER 9
Periodization

Cancer care unfolds in phases: the lead-up to surgery, cycles of chemotherapy or immunotherapy, courses of radiation, rehabilitation, and survivorship. Each phase brings its own physical and psychological demands. A "one speed" exercise plan will fit some days and fail on others. That is the first truth of periodization: we plan ahead, then we adapt.

Periodization began in elite sport, but its value in oncology has nothing to do with imitating athletes. It is the logic of sequencing stress and recovery—when to push, when to hold, and when to change direction—so the right stimulus arrives at the right time. In oncology, the "big events" aren't races; they are surgery dates, infusion days, radiation fractions, scan weeks, neurological flares, and milestones in recovery. The plan bends around these anchors, not the other way around.

If that sounds complex, it is. But complex does not need to be confusing. In this chapter, I explain the moving parts that make periodization work in cancer care: the planning models we rely on, the way we sequence training stresses, how we pair nutrition and psychological support with training phases, and the simple monitoring that protects consistency even when symptoms fluctuate. Think of this chapter as a map—not fixed, but living—designed for a landscape that keeps shifting.

Why Periodization Matters in Cancer Care

A useful starting point is the **fitness–fatigue paradigm**. Every exercise session produces two effects at once: it creates fatigue now and fitness later. If the next session comes too soon, fatigue accumulates faster than fitness and performance drifts downward. If we wait too long, capacity decays before we can progress. Periodization is the method by which we arrange these waves so that, over weeks and months, the trend is upward rather than chaotic.

Cancer care adds an additional layer: treatment-related fatigue is irregular and often intense. Chemotherapy may flatten you for two or three days and then lift. Radiation tends to create a slow, cumulative drag. Immunotherapy can produce unpredictable fluctuations. Steroid therapy may cause fluid shifts, blood sugar instability, insomnia, and muscle catabolism. Periodization lets us match training to these rhythms and preserve the gains you fight for.

In one sentence: Plan phases ahead, then autoregulate day to day based on symptoms, side effects, and recovery—so training fits you rather than forcing you to fit the training.

The Moving Parts

Periodization in oncology is a systems puzzle. Several domains interact:

- **Treatment calendar** (surgery, infusion days, radiation fractions)
- **Physiological response** (fitness rising gradually; fatigue rising quickly and falling unpredictably)
- **Training content** (strength, hypertrophy, power, aerobic conditioning, balance, bone loading)
- **Medical realities** (bone density, neuropathy, lymphedema risk, comorbidities)
- **Life logistics** (childcare, travel, clinic hours, finances)
- **Psychology** (mood, anxiety, cognition, motivation)
- **Nutrition** (fuel availability, appetite, GI tolerance)

A good plan anticipates the fixed components—like surgery dates—and flexes around the variable ones—like nausea after an infusion. There is no single "correct" periodized plan; there is only the correct process for arriving at the **next plan**.

Two Practical Periodization Models

Many periodization styles exist in sport science, but in oncology two models consistently prove useful: **parallel periodization** and **emphasis periodization**. Both rely on the resistance and aerobic training principles described in Chapters 4–6; here we focus on *when* and *how* these tools appear across a training block.

1. Parallel Periodization

Parallel periodization trains several physical qualities—such as strength, hypertrophy, and aerobic fitness—at the same time. The emphasis is balanced, and the "dials" of volume, intensity, and frequency move gradually across weeks.

This approach suits:

- people rebuilding general fitness
- those newer to structured training
- patients with fluctuating energy
- most prehabilitation phases

Because the load is spread across systems, it avoids overtaxing any single one.

Example
A woman preparing for lumpectomy completes two full-body strength sessions per week (one hypertrophy-oriented, one strength-oriented), plus three aerobic sessions (two steady MICT sessions and one short interval session). Intensity rises gradually over four weeks. On low-energy days, we trim sets or volume but keep the rhythm—because consistency wins over perfection.

2. Emphasis Periodization

In emphasis periodization, one quality—such as strength, aerobic fitness, or bone loading—is the priority for a few weeks, while other qualities are maintained at a lower dose. Emphasis blocks are shifted over time.

This approach suits:

- people with a clear primary goal (e.g., bone protection on ADT, raising aerobic capacity leading up to surgery)
- those requiring careful sequencing to minimise **interference** (see Chapter 5)
- survivorship training with longer-term aims

Example

A man on androgen deprivation therapy begins with an emphasis on strength: two focused lifting sessions and two short aerobic sessions per week. After eight weeks he has regained sufficient muscular capacity to begin tiny doses of impact loading. We keep one strength session heavy and gradually nudge aerobic sessions upward to help with weight control—rotating emphasis block by block.

Both models rely heavily on **autoregulation**—adapting the day's training to your current symptoms, sleep, mood, and recovery capacity. RPE, RIR, and simple symptom check-ins (see Chapter 4) allow a structured plan to remain humane and adaptable.

The Building Blocks Inside a Session (Applied to Periodization)

In Chapters 4, 5, and 6 I explain the technical details of strength, hypertrophy, power, aerobic conditioning, balance training, and session spacing. Here, we focus solely on how these tools are **sequenced over time**.

Strength and Hypertrophy

Muscle supports treatment tolerance, metabolism, and functional independence. Across a periodized plan, we adjust:

- **volume** (sets and exercises)
- **intensity** (load and RIR)
- **tempo**
- **set structures** (straight sets, ascending, descending, pyramids, supersets)
- **rest intervals**

Hypertrophy-oriented work (≈6–12 reps, 2–3 RIR) appears consistently across blocks because muscle mass provides foundational medicine. We vary the emphasis and volume but rarely remove hypertrophy entirely.

Cluster sets, accentuated eccentric work, and machine-based options (see Chapter 5) are introduced strategically—often during chemotherapy, fatigue spikes, or phases requiring high quality with lower cardiovascular strain.

Power and Function

Power is layered on top of strength once control and tolerance are established. Periodized plans introduce:

- low-load medicine ball throws
- controlled, quicker sit-to-stands
- step-ups with a deliberate drive
- leg press with rapid concentric phase

These are typically added in mid-to-late blocks, not at the beginning of treatment, and never during periods of uncontrolled symptoms.

Bone Loading

Impact training is introduced only after a foundation of strength is built (usually 6–12 weeks). The periodized sequence is:

1. Strength first
2. Low-level impact (heel drops)
3. Progression to small hops or jumps (if appropriate, cleared, and symptom-free)

For patients with bone metastases, we follow conservative protocols described in the bone chapter and avoid impact entirely. Periodization here means carefully **phasing** what is safe and appropriate—not pushing impact arbitrarily.

Aerobic Conditioning

Chapters 4 and 6 explain aerobic training in depth. Within a periodized plan, we time aerobic sessions to support—not compete with—strength work. On high-fatigue days, interval training with short bursts and ample recovery may be easier than long continuous sessions. On more stable days, longer MICT sessions build endurance.

Balance and Stability

Balance elements appear lightly in early blocks and are expanded as strength and confidence improve. We avoid unstable-surface training that adds risk without meaningful benefit; instead, we progress single-leg tasks, trunk control, and ground-based movements over time.

Session Spacing and Splits

Strength sessions targeting the same muscle groups require ~48 hours between them. Total-body training two to three times per week works well early in treatment. As capacity grows—or when training four or more days per week—we shift to **upper/lower** or **push/pull** splits to distribute fatigue and support higher weekly volume.

Variety Across Blocks

Variety prevents stagnation and maintains engagement. Ascending sets, descending sets, pyramids, and supersets (see Chapter 5) are introduced across blocks—not every week—to create fresh stimuli without overwhelming recovery.

Periodization Across the Cancer Continuum

Prehabilitation (Before Surgery)

Goal: arrive at surgery with greater fitness, strength, and resilience.

Prehabilitation focuses on whole-body strength, aerobic capacity, mobility, and recovery habits. Even 4–8 weeks make a measurable difference.

Example plan

- **Weeks 1–2:** two full-body strength sessions (one hypertrophy-focused, one strength-focused); 2–3 aerobic sessions (20–30 minutes steady, plus one short interval session); daily range of motion (flexibility) and mobility exercise.
- **Weeks 3–4:** maintain frequency; add 5–10 minutes to aerobic sessions; increase one set on major lifts; add a small amount of cluster work to maintain quality.
- **Final week:** taper—reduce volume 20–40%, keep intensity moderate, maintain routine but avoid fatigue.

Nutrition (discussed fully in the nutrition chapter) supports this block with protein-forward meals, hydration, and stable energy intake.

Chemotherapy (Example Two-Week Microcycle)

Goal: protect muscle and fitness, dissipate side-effects, manage unpredictable fatigue, and align with the infusion rhythm.

We often use a two-week "wave" linked to each chemotherapy cycle:

- **Days 1–3 post-infusion:** 10–20 minutes easy walking, mobility, light resistance exercise.
- **Days 4–10:** one interval aerobic session, one steady MICT session (25–35 minutes), and one full-body strength session at moderate reps.
- **Days 11–14:** taper volume slightly; keep moving but leave a set in reserve.

Short pre-infusion aerobic bouts may help perfusion if cleared by the oncology team.

Radiation Therapy

Goal: support tissue oxygenation, enhance effectiveness, maintain strength, and manage cumulative fatigue.

We maintain strength at a conservative dose (high quality, lower volume) and emphasize regular aerobic work. Short, steady sessions or interval training at moderate intensity often fit best. With supervision, a brief pre-fraction bout is desirable if possible as exercise priming.

Immunotherapy

Goal: support immune function and preserve muscle while adapting to variable side effects.

Two strength sessions per week can maintain muscle effectively. Aerobic sessions are flexible. Autoregulation is crucial because symptom patterns vary between individuals and over cycles. An extensive example is provided in a later chapter.

Steroid Therapy

Goal: counteract catabolic effects on muscle and bone, manage blood sugar and weight, and protect mood and sleep.

We emphasize hypertrophy-oriented strength, balanced nutrition, and aerobic activity that supports glycemic control. Impact and balance elements are added gradually based on bone status.

Survivorship

Goal: enhance cardiorespiratory fitness, muscular strength and mass, metabolic control, and bone health in ways that support long-term function, reduce recurrence risk, and lower the likelihood of developing other chronic diseases.

We may rotate emphasis blocks across the year: bone-focused strength and impact, aerobic capacity, power, or higher-volume hypertrophy. Survivorship training applies periodization to longer horizons, allowing progressive development of cardiovascular, musculoskeletal, and metabolic capacity beyond the constraints of active treatment.

Nutrition Periodization: Fueling the Plan

Training is the signal; nutrition is the building material. The specifics of protein, energy balance, glycemic control, and dietary patterns are covered in the nutrition chapter. Periodization here refers to **timing nutrition with training load and treatment cycles**:

- **Prehabilitation:** adequate protein across the day, nutrient-rich food quality, hydration, and—when appropriate—focused weight management.
- **Chemotherapy:** match intake to fluctuating appetite; use small, frequent, protein-rich meals; on stronger days, fuel training with a bit more energy.
- **Radiation:** emphasize hydration and tissue-repair nutrients; adjust textures for oral discomfort.
- **Steroids:** distribute carbohydrates thoughtfully, maintain steady protein intake.
- **Fat loss phases (where appropriate):** increase aerobic volume gradually and maintain hypertrophy-oriented lifting to protect muscle.

The key is alignment: harder training days receive more energy and protein; recovery days emphasize quality and consistency.

Psychological Strategies—Also Periodized

Psychological factors influence exercise tolerance, adherence, and recovery throughout cancer treatment and survivorship. We align psychological supports with treatment phases:

- **Before surgery or new treatment:** brief daily breathing practices, goal setting, and sleep support.
- **During treatment:** pacing strategies, tiny routines for low-energy days, social support, and supervised group sessions.
- **In survivorship:** resilience-building, graded physical challenges, and goal-directed planning for long-term exercise adherence.

These strategies maintain consistency when motivation fluctuates, and they help exercise feel purposeful rather than burdensome.

Monitoring and Autoregulation—Simple Tools That Hold the Plan Together

Autoregulation allows a periodized program to adjust appropriately to day-to-day variations in symptoms, recovery, and treatment effects. Tools include:

- **RPE (0–10):** target ranges instead of exact numbers.
- **Reps in Reserve:** stop with 1–3 reps left; on hard days, leave more in the tank.
- **Traffic light readiness:**
    - **Green:** symptoms stable → follow the plan.
    - **Yellow:** poor sleep, mild nausea, unusual soreness → trim volume; keep intensity moderate; use cluster sets or machine-based options.
    - **Red:** fever, dizziness, new bone pain, uncontrolled symptoms → stop and contact your medical team.

- **Session order:** strength first, then aerobic work (or separate sessions), to protect strength and bone goals.
- **Weekly reflection:** note what worked and one change to improve the next week.

The 20% Rule

On days you feel unexpectedly strong, cap increases to no more than **20% more volume** than planned. On harder days, doing **something**—even 10 minutes—maintains the habit loop and eases the return to full training.

Safety Anchors Across Periodization

Detailed safety guidance appears in earlier chapters; here we highlight the periodization-specific implications:

- **Bone health:** Impact loading is introduced only after a strength base is established (6–12 weeks). In bone metastases or high-risk sites, avoid impact entirely and use the conservative protocols described in the bone chapter.
- **Lymphedema:** Progressive resistance training is safe. Progress gradually and monitor for changes; see the lymphedema chapter for details.
- **Warm-up and cool-down:** Smooth transitions reduce adverse events and help heart rate and blood pressure adjust appropriately—especially when switching between upper and lower body work.
- **Red flag symptoms:** chest pain, new bone pain, sudden breathlessness, fever or neutropenic risk, neurological symptoms → stop immediately and seek guidance.

These anchors ensure that periodized plans remain safe and sustainable.

Three Extended Case Studies

Case 1 (Wei) — Eight Weeks to Surgery (Stage III Lung Cancer)

Goals: raise aerobic capacity, build strength, reduce excess body fat and systemic inflammation, enhance surgical resilience.

Starting point: low fitness, minimal training history.

Plan (parallel model):

- **Weeks 1–4:**
    - Strength twice weekly: one hypertrophy-oriented, one strength-oriented.
    - Aerobic: two MICT sessions building from ~25 minutes, plus one brief interval training session.
    - Variety through ascending sets and small cluster doses when fatigue rises.
- **Weeks 5–8:**
    - Maintain frequency; add one set to main lifts; extend MICT to ~40 minutes; increase intervals intensity to HIIT as tolerated.
    - Final week: reduce volume 25–40% to taper while keeping intensity.

Why it works: Aerobic capacity and strength both predict post-operative outcomes; entering surgery physiologically "loaded" improves recovery.

Case 2 (Fatima) — Six Chemotherapy Infusions Over 12 Weeks (Stage III Colorectal)

Goals: maintain fitness, manage fatigue, support treatment tolerance, enhance treatment effectiveness.

Starting point: low fitness, cancer-related fatigue, no resistance training history.

Plan (emphasis model tied to infusion rhythm):

- **Non-infusion week:**
    - Aerobic (2–3 sessions): one HIIT session (RPE 6–7), one or two steady 25–35 minute walks/cycles.
    - Strength: one full-body session (moderate load, 10–12 reps × 2–3 sets).
- **Infusion week:**
    - Two short sessions (20–30 minutes): light aerobic plus cluster-style strength (e.g., leg press and row at 2+2+2+2).

Why it works: By matching the peaks and troughs of the infusion cycle, the plan protects adaptations without provoking crashes.

Case 3 (Yasmin) — Two Years Post-Chemo, on Hormone Therapy (Breast Cancer, Low BMD)

Goals: rebuild muscle and bone density, return to recreational running.
Starting point: recreationally active, low BMD, peripheral neuropathy.

Plan (emphasis blocks):

- **Block 1 (5 weeks):** two strength sessions (one hypertrophy, one strength), one MICT session, one HIIT session.
- **Block 2 (5 weeks):** introduce low-level impact; extend MICT to 45 minutes.
- **Block 3 (5 weeks):** heavier strength work (4–6 reps), progressive impact if pain-free, longer MICT sessions.

Why it works: Strength prepares the tissues for impact; impact provides the bone-specific stimulus; and aerobic conditioning supports her running goals. Sequencing the blocks prevents overload, respects her low bone mineral density, and rebuilds confidence step by step.

Putting It All Together: A Living Plan

Periodization is the art of sequencing—not a rigid calendar. We plan **microcycles** (1–2 weeks), **mesocycles** (4–8 weeks), and **macrocycles**

(3–12 months). We select a parallel or emphasis model based on your medical status, your goals, and your energy profile. Inside each session, we choose tools—volume, tempo, rest intervals, exercise order, accentuated eccentric, cluster sets—not randomly, but with intent that matches the phase you are in.

We then align nutrition to support the training load, use psychological strategies to sustain motivation, and monitor symptoms and recovery to guide autoregulation. The result is a plan that moves with you rather than against you.

Checklist — Starting a Periodized Plan

- Get clearance from your oncology and exercise team; share any new bone pain or neurological symptoms.
- Identify your anchor events (surgery date, infusion days, radiation schedule) and plan outward from them.
- Choose a model: **parallel** if you need balanced conditioning; **emphasis** if you have a clear priority (bone, strength, aerobic capacity).
- Set two achievable process goals for the month (e.g., "two strength sessions per week" or "three 20-minute walks").
- Decide which autoregulation tools you will use (RPE, RIR, traffic-light readiness) and what adjustments you will make on yellow or red days.
- Align nutrition with training (more protein and energy on heavier days; hydration and steady intake on low days).
- Add one simple recovery habit (five minutes of breathing in the evening or walking after dinner).

Checklist — Chemotherapy Microcycle (2 Weeks)

Chemotherapy cycles naturally create a periodization cycle in training. The principles below outline how to structure training across a typical chemotherapy cycle to align with expected physiological fluctuations. This can then be adjusted for longer or shorter cycles.

- **Days 1–3 (Post-infusion: recovery-focused)**
  - Keep sessions short and low volume.
  - Gentle walking (10–20 minutes), mobility, or very light resistance work.
  - Prioritise symptom monitoring, hydration, and sleep.
  - Use machine-based, body weight or bands, regressed as needed, or omit resistance training if too difficult.
- **Days 4–10 (Mid-cycle: highest training capacity)**
  - One interval-based aerobic session (short bursts of effort with adequate recovery).
  - One steady moderate-intensity session (25–35 minutes).
  - Two full-body strength sessions using moderate (8-12 RM) loads and leaving 2–3 reps in reserve.
  - Volume is increased cautiously based on symptoms.
- **Days 11–14 (Pre-infusion: consolidate and taper)**
  - Continue exercise intensity but reduce volume by ~20–30%.
  - Short steady aerobic sessions or brief strength sessions with lower volume load.
  - Leave an additional set or rep "in the tank."
  - Prioritise sleep, hydration, and maintaining routine.

On low-energy days at any point: Short "exercise snacks" (two or three 5–10 minute bouts) are effective and often better tolerated than a continuous session. Protein and fluid intake should remain consistent across the cycle.

Lymphedema Considerations

For people with or at risk of lymphedema, progressive resistance training is safe when introduced gradually and monitored appropriately. Compression garments may be used when recommended. Training loads are advanced cautiously, and any changes in limb symptoms should be reviewed. Detailed guidance is provided in the lymphedema chapter.

Closing Thoughts

Periodization provides a structured way to organise training across the changing demands of cancer treatment and recovery. It allows exercise intensity, volume, and frequency to be matched to predictable treatment cycles and day-to-day variations in symptoms and readiness.

When applied well, periodization supports improvements in cardiorespiratory fitness, muscle mass, strength, bone health, and metabolic function. It helps patients approach key treatment events—such as surgery or infusions—with better physiological capacity and facilitates recovery afterwards. Rather than promoting constant progression, periodization highlights the importance of selecting an appropriate training dose for each day and adjusting the plan as clinical circumstances change.

CHAPTER 10

Cancer, Treatments, and Bone Loss

Bone health is a quiet problem for many people living with cancer. Fatigue, nausea, and pain usually make themselves known. Bone loss often does not. It can progress silently for years until the first fracture appears, and by that point the damage is already done—a broken hip, a collapsed vertebra, or a rib fracture that refuses to heal properly. These events are not minor interruptions in life. They can lead to long-term disability, loss of independence, and reduced survival.

The risk of bone loss is highest in people receiving hormone-suppressing therapies such as androgen deprivation therapy for prostate cancer or aromatase inhibitors for breast cancer. These therapies remain essential for controlling disease, but they accelerate the loss of bone at the spine, hip and other vulnerable sites. Many people are also older when treatment begins, and age-related bone loss is already underway. Cancer, treatment, and age can combine to weaken the skeleton and increase the risk of falls, fractures, and frailty.

The encouraging part of this story is that exercise medicine offers powerful tools to protect bone. While we cannot fully prevent bone loss for everyone, we can slow it, stabilize it, and sometimes improve bone strength. The key is specificity. Bones respond only when mechanical signals reach a certain threshold. Walking is excellent for fatigue, cardiovascular health, and mood, but it does not deliver enough force to stimulate bone. To genuinely strengthen bone, we rely on resistance training and impact-based movements that deliver the loading characteristics bones are designed to respond to.

In this chapter, I explain why bones weaken during and after cancer treatment, how different therapies accelerate bone loss, and how exercise can be used as a frontline therapy. I describe the types of exercise that are most effective, how to use them safely, and what this means for people living with or beyond cancer.

Why Bones Weaken in Cancer and Its Treatments

The Natural Course of Bone Ageing

Bone is living tissue. Throughout life it undergoes constant remodeling as bone-building and bone-resorbing cells work together to maintain structure. In youth, bone formation slightly exceeds bone breakdown. As we move through midlife and older age, this balance begins to shift.

For women, bone loss accelerates after menopause when estrogen levels fall. Estrogen helps slow bone breakdown and supports the maintenance of healthy bone tissue. For men, testosterone contributes to bone formation and muscle mass, and its gradual decline with age also weakens the skeleton. By the time many people reach their sixties or seventies, their bones are naturally thinner and more fragile than in earlier decades.

The Impact of Cancer Therapies

Cancer treatments often amplify this natural process.

In men with prostate cancer, androgen deprivation therapy lowers testosterone and estrogen to extremely low levels. Within months, measurable bone loss occurs at the spine and hip. If this continues over years, fracture risk increases significantly, particularly for vertebral and hip fractures—both associated with reduced survival and long-term loss of independence.

Women treated for hormone receptor–positive breast cancer often receive aromatase inhibitors, which block estrogen production almost entirely. Without estrogen's protective effect, bone resorption increases and the spine, hip, and wrist commonly thin at a faster rate. Chemotherapy and corticosteroids may add further strain by impairing bone-forming cells and altering calcium regulation.

Radiotherapy can weaken bone in a more localized way. High radiation doses affect bone marrow, disrupt the blood supply that nourishes bone, and directly damage the cells responsible for bone turnover. Areas such as the pelvis, spine, and ribs may become more vulnerable to fracture months or even years after treatment.

In advanced cancer, bone metastases erode bone from within, creating weak regions at risk of pathological fracture.

The Compounding Effect of Inactivity

Activity levels often drop during cancer treatment. Fatigue, pain, low mood, and uncertainty about what is safe can all reduce movement. With less weight-bearing activity and fewer strong muscle contractions, bones receive fewer mechanical signals to maintain their density. Muscles then weaken, further reducing loading on the skeleton. This can create a cycle of weakness, instability, and increased risk of falls.

The Consequences of Bone Loss

Bone loss is not just a change in a DEXA scan. It has profound real-world consequences.

Vertebral and hip fractures are particularly serious. They often require hospitalization, surgery, or prolonged rehabilitation. Many people never fully regain their previous function. Spinal fractures can cause chronic pain, loss of height, and a forward-bent posture that affects breathing and digestion.

Fear of falling is common after a fracture or a close call. People begin to avoid activities they once enjoyed, move less, and lose more strength and balance. This avoidance ironically increases the chance of another fall. Large studies show that fractures in people with cancer are associated with increased mortality, especially within the first year after a hip fracture.

Bone health is therefore not simply a structural issue—it is central to maintaining independence, confidence, and long-term wellbeing.

Why Exercise Is a Bone Medicine

Bones respond to mechanical forces. When muscles contract and ground forces travel through the legs, hips, and spine, osteocytes sense the mechanical strain. These cells act as sensors and communicate with bone-building and bone-resorbing cells to adjust bone structure. This process—mechanotransduction—is how bones interpret physical loading and decide whether they need to reinforce themselves.

The forces must be large enough or rapid enough to be recognized. Gentle movements and slow walking generate forces below the threshold required to stimulate bone, which is why they do not maintain or increase bone density. By contrast, resistance training provides heavy, controlled loading through major bones and joints, and impact loading provides quick, high-force signals that bones respond to very efficiently.

Exercise also strengthens the entire system around the skeleton. Strong muscles support joints, protect against falls, and improve alignment. Better balance and coordination reduce the likelihood of tripping. Exercise improves metabolic health and reduces inflammation, contributing to a healthier environment for bone.

Together, these effects create a more resilient body even when bone density improves only modestly.

What the Evidence Shows

Clinical trials and systematic reviews in exercise oncology consistently show that:

Men on androgen deprivation therapy do not maintain bone mass with aerobic exercise alone or with low-intensity resistance training. Only programs that combine heavy resistance training with impact loading have been shown to slow bone loss at the spine and hip.

Women on aromatase inhibitors respond similarly. Supervised resistance training improves lumbar spine bone density, and the benefit is greater when simple impact exercises such as heel drops, stamping, or gentle jumps are included. Walking programs alone, even when performed regularly, do not influence bone density.

People with bone metastases can safely perform resistance training when programs are designed and supervised by experienced oncology exercise professionals. Studies show that bone density in metastatic vertebrae can be maintained and sometimes improved when direct heavy loading of affected regions is avoided.

Across studies, the central conclusion is clear: exercise protects bone only when it includes targeted mechanical loading.

Exercise Strategies for Bone Health in Cancer

Resistance Training

Resistance training is the foundation of exercise for bone health. Multi-joint exercises such as squats, leg presses, deadlifts, chest presses, and rows deliver substantial loading through major bones and joints. These exercises also build the muscle strength needed to protect against falls.

A practical approach is to begin with loads that feel challenging by the final few repetitions of a set and gradually increase resistance as technique improves. Many people work with two to four sets of eight to twelve repetitions per exercise. When performed two or three times each week, this provides a strong osteogenic stimulus.

A foundation phase of resistance training over one to three months allows muscles, tendons, and joints to adapt before introducing more rapid loading patterns.

Impact Loading

Impact exercises create quick, high-force signals that bones respond to efficiently. These include heel drops, light stamping, small jumps, or hops. The goal is crisp, controlled contact rather than height or speed.

This is where hormone-suppressing therapies require specific attention. Men starting androgen deprivation therapy and women beginning aromatase inhibitors experience accelerated bone loss from the moment treatment starts. Waiting several months before sending a bone-loading signal allows bone loss to accumulate. For this reason, it is important to begin bone-targeted exercise at the same time as the therapy begins.

However, this does not mean jumping into high-impact exercise immediately. People still require the strength, joint control, and technical foundations that resistance training builds. The solution is to begin traditional resistance training and introduce very low-level impact loading at the same time. Light stamping, small controlled heel drops, or gentle step-downs provide early mechanical signals without excessive stress. These exercises can be progressed gradually as strength and confidence improve.

Combined Programs

The strongest outcomes come from programs that combine resistance training with some level of impact loading. In men on androgen deprivation therapy, this combination is the only approach shown to slow bone loss at both the spine and hip. Aerobic plus resistance training improves fitness and fatigue but does not protect bone unless bone-targeted loading is included.

In practice, resistance training forms the base, while short bursts of impact or modified impact provide additional mechanical signaling.

Aerobic Exercise

Aerobic exercise remains an essential part of overall cancer care. Walking, cycling, and swimming improve cardiovascular health, manage fatigue, support metabolic function, and enhance mood. These benefits are substantial.

However, aerobic training generates forces below the threshold required to stimulate bone. It is therefore a complement to, not a substitute for, resistance and impact loading.

Safety in Bone Metastases

When bone metastases are present, exercise must be adapted carefully. The aim is to maintain strength and balance while avoiding excessive loading through affected sites. High-impact exercises and heavy loading of metastatic regions are avoided, but resistance training for unaffected areas remains both safe and beneficial.

Supervision by an accredited exercise professional with oncology experience is essential. Knowledge of the exact location and extent of bone involvement guides safe program design and helps avoid unnecessary restrictions.

Designing a Practical Program

A practical program for someone at risk of treatment-related bone loss typically includes two or three resistance training sessions each week. These sessions target major muscle groups with exercises performed for several sets of controlled repetitions, gradually increasing resistance over time.

Short bouts of impact or modified impact—such as heel drops, light stamping, or controlled jumps—are integrated on most resistance days. Early volumes may be as low as ten to twenty contacts, increasing as technique improves.

Balance and mobility work is performed throughout the week. Single-leg stands, slow tandem walking, and dynamic stretching support joint mobility and reduce fall risk.

Aerobic exercise is included on most days for twenty to forty minutes. Many people choose brisk walking, cycling, or treadmill work, adjusting intensity to match energy levels and treatment side effects.

Programs are always tailored to individual diagnosis, treatment phase, bone density, fracture history, and other medical conditions.

Beyond Bone Density: Functional Protection

Bone density scans tell only part of the story. Many fractures occur in people who do not meet the criteria for osteoporosis. Real fracture risk comes from a combination of somewhat thin bones, weak muscles, impaired balance, and increased likelihood of falling.

Exercise addresses all these factors. Strength training builds powerful legs and hips. Impact loading stimulates bone. Balance work sharpens stability and reaction time. Perhaps most importantly, regular training builds confidence in exercise. People who train consistently fall less often, and when they do stumble, they are more capable of recovering.

This functional protection is one of the most important contributions exercise makes to bone health.

Hormone-Suppressing Therapies: A Narrative Comparison

Women taking aromatase inhibitors and men receiving androgen deprivation therapy experience parallel patterns of accelerated bone and muscle loss, although the hormonal mechanisms differ. In women, near-complete suppression of estrogen accelerates bone breakdown and often causes joint pain, stiffness, hot flushes, and shifts in body composition. Exercise priorities include preserving bone density, maintaining lean mass, easing stiffness, and supporting cardiovascular and mental health. Moderate to heavy resistance training is central, with short periods of low-level impact added early to stimulate bone. Aerobic exercise supports metabolic and emotional health, while mobility work reduces the joint discomfort that many women experience on aromatase inhibitors.

Men on androgen deprivation therapy experience a profound fall in testosterone, leading to rapid losses in muscle and bone, increased fat mass, and impaired glucose and lipid regulation. Many men feel as if their bodies have aged dramatically within weeks. Resistance training is again the cornerstone of therapy. By targeting the large muscles of the legs, back, and chest, men can preserve or even regain lean mass despite low testosterone. Where safe, impact loading provides an important signal for bone. Aerobic work—sometimes including intervals—helps improve metabolic health and maintain energy. A high-protein Mediterranean-style dietary pattern complements training by supporting muscle repair and stabilizing blood sugar and cholesterol.

In both groups, exercise provides a sense of agency at a time when many feel physically vulnerable. Combined with medical therapies such as calcium, vitamin D, and bone-protective medications, exercise can shift the trajectory from steep decline to maintenance or improvement.

Conclusion

Bone loss is one of the hidden but significant consequences of cancer and its treatments. People receiving hormone-suppressing therapies, older adults, and those with advanced disease all face accelerated skeletal decline that can undermine independence and shorten life.

Exercise medicine is one of the most effective countermeasures available. To protect bone, exercise must be specific. Bones respond best to heavy resistance training and appropriately dosed impact loading. When delivered safely and progressively, this combination preserves bone density, strengthens muscle, improves balance, reduces falls, and maintains mobility.

The message is clear: exercise is not simply safe for bones—it is essential. It belongs alongside medical treatments, supplements, and ongoing monitoring as a standard part of cancer care. Protecting bone health means protecting mobility, autonomy, and long-term wellbeing, and exercise is one of the most powerful tools we have to achieve that.

CHAPTER 11
Impact Loading

Impact loading is a powerful and highly targeted method to slow—and in some cases partially reverse—loss of bone. Bone loss during cancer treatment can occur for several reasons: reduced physical activity, periods of unloading after surgery or illness, medication side effects, and the direct or indirect effects of cancer itself. Hormone-suppressing treatments for breast and prostate cancer accelerate this process further, causing rapid declines in bone mass and structural integrity. Without intervention, these changes can compromise mobility, increase fracture risk, and reduce independence.

Traditional resistance training is effective for maintaining or improving bone in many healthy older adults and can significantly slow bone loss during menopause. However, resistance training alone is often insufficient for people undergoing profound hormone suppression—such as aromatase inhibitor therapy or androgen deprivation therapy. In these situations, bone requires an additional, more specific mechanical signal.

Impact loading provides that signal. It delivers rapid, high-rate changes in force that bone cells are particularly sensitive to. Osteoblasts and osteocytes respond most strongly to brief, sharp increases in mechanical load rather than steady or slow forces. For this reason, impact training uses controlled drills that generate short, crisp spikes in ground reaction forces. The aim is always safe, technically sound impact that is scaled to the individual.

Preparing for Impact Training

A preparatory strength phase of eight to twelve weeks is ideal for most people before progressing to higher-intensity impact training. Resistance training builds the muscular strength and joint stability needed to tolerate impact safely. Individuals who have already been engaged in resistance training can often begin impact work sooner.

When bone loss is accelerating rapidly—such as in the first months after starting androgen deprivation therapy or aromatase inhibitors—it is not advisable to delay impact work entirely. In these cases, resistance training begins immediately and is paired with very low-intensity impact drills. Light stamping, controlled heel drops, or small step-downs provide an early mechanical signal while strength and mobility are being restored.

Safety, symptom monitoring, and gradual progression remain central throughout. Strength and impact develop in parallel, with impact introduced only as tolerated.

Footwear and Surfaces

Footwear significantly influences how much force reaches the skeleton. Highly cushioned running shoes disperse impact, lowering the loading rate that bone cells respond to. This is desirable for long-distance running but counterproductive when the goal is to stimulate bone.

For low-intensity impact exercises—marching, light stamping, or small jumps—bare feet or firm, minimally cushioned shoes can enhance the osteogenic signal. However, this is not appropriate for everyone. Pre-existing foot problems, neuropathy, balance concerns, and joint issues may require more supportive footwear. In all cases, safety is the priority.

Impact training should be performed on stable, non-slip surfaces such as carpet, a firm exercise mat, wood, or vinyl flooring. Uneven or slippery surfaces increase injury risk and should be avoided.

Impact Loading Exercises: A Controlled Progression

The following progression moves from gentle to more advanced exercises. Most people will benefit substantially from the early and intermediate levels; progression is not mandatory and should always reflect symptoms, conditioning, and confidence.

Marching on the Spot

Begin by lifting each knee in a controlled manner and placing the foot down with a firm, deliberate contact. As control improves, the landing can become slightly crisper to introduce a clearer mechanical signal. For many people, this level provides adequate stimulus and can be maintained long-term.

Heel Drops

Rise onto the toes and drop onto the heels with a controlled, decisive landing. This produces a rapid upward-travelling signal through the legs, pelvis, and spine. The speed of the descent determines the loading rate.

Vertical Jumps

From a comfortable stance, perform a small squat and jump vertically, landing softly with control. Jumps can be performed singly or in short sequences. Individuals with balance concerns may hold a stable support.

Skipping in Place

Skipping introduces periods of single-leg loading. It can be performed on the spot or over short distances. The alternating pattern increases mechanical load through the supporting leg.

Hopping

Perform small hops on one leg, then switch sides. This increases both impact and balance demands. Light support from a rail or bench may be used as needed.

Drop Jumps

Begin from a low step (15–30 cm). Step off, land on both feet, briefly absorb the landing, and then immediately jump vertically. Dropping from height increases landing velocity and therefore impact load.

Hurdle Jumps

Low, flexible hurdles are arranged in a straight line. Using a double-leg bounding motion, clear each hurdle with short contacts between them. The hurdles are designed to tip easily to reduce trip risk.

Bounding

A highly advanced drill involving long, exaggerated strides over 10–15 meters, generating high loads through the legs and pelvis. Only individuals with excellent strength, coordination, and conditioning progress to this level.

Structuring an Impact Training Session

Impact exercises are ballistic, so a thorough warm-up is essential. Three to five minutes of walking on the spot, step-ups, light squats, and gentle lunges prepare joints, tendons, and muscles for higher loading rates.

After the warm-up, beginners typically start with marching on the spot, performing 5–10 impacts per leg. During and after the session, attention is paid to joint comfort. The following day is an important checkpoint: any sustained joint pain, swelling, or deep bone discomfort signals the need to reduce intensity or volume.

Impact adaptation occurs quickly. Sessions of 10–15 minutes are usually sufficient. A total of 60–120 impacts is typical for a full session, though beginners start far below this. Quality and control are more important than volume.

Progression and Weekly Frequency

Progression involves gradually increasing repetitions, sets, or the challenge level of exercises. Many people begin with one set of marching and gradually increase to two or three sets of 10 contacts. Once this is comfortable, a second exercise—such as heel drops or skipping—can be introduced.

The body's response determines the pace of progression. If exercises feel smooth and controlled without excessive soreness, the next step may be attempted. If discomfort occurs, the program is scaled back.

Most individuals begin with two or three impact sessions per week, spaced at least 48 hours apart. As conditioning improves, training may increase to three or four sessions per week. A small number of people with high capacity may reach five sessions, though this is not required for bone health.

Periodizing impact across the week—higher intensity on one day, lower on another, and moderate on a third—helps manage fatigue and reduce injury risk. Splitting sessions into morning and afternoon blocks can also improve quality and maintain control.

Program Structure: Beginner, Intermediate, Advanced

Impact loading is one area where clear stages are clinically useful because the mechanical demands increase quickly and require careful progression.

Beginners

- **Repetitions per set:** 4–8
- **Sets per exercise:** 1–2
- **Exercises per session:** 1–3
- **Typical exercises:** marching, heel drops, small vertical jumps
- **Frequency:** 2–3 sessions/week with rest days between

Intermediate

- **Repetitions per set:** 6–12
- **Sets per exercise:** 2–3
- **Exercises per session:** 2–3
- **Typical exercises:** heel drops, vertical jumps, skipping, hopping
- **Frequency:** 3–4 sessions/week

Advanced

- **Repetitions per set:** 10–15
- **Sets per exercise:** 3
- **Exercises per session:** 3–4

- **Typical exercises:** hopping, drop jumps, hurdle jumps, bounding
- **Frequency:** up to 5 sessions/week depending on recovery

At all levels, varying exercises across the week and occasionally returning to lower-intensity drills improves quality and reduces overload.

Notes on Progression

Impact training requires close monitoring of symptoms. Pain, swelling, or deep bone discomfort indicates the need to reduce load or regress temporarily. Varying exercises and dividing sessions into shorter blocks can maintain quality while reducing risk.

Safety and Professional Guidance

Impact training is potent and must be applied carefully. People with significant osteoporosis, previous fragility fractures, or bone metastases require individualized assessment. In these cases, guidance from an accredited exercise professional with oncology expertise is essential. Even when high-impact drills are contraindicated, modified impact and targeted strength training can still provide meaningful benefit.

Conclusion

Impact loading adds an essential dimension to bone-focused exercise medicine. Resistance training builds the strength and joint stability required to support the skeleton; impact drills provide the rapid mechanical signals that bone cells respond to most strongly. Together, they help slow or partially reverse treatment-related bone loss.

Most individuals will remain within the early and intermediate levels, which provide substantial benefit when performed consistently. Marching with firm contacts, heel drops, simple jumps, and—when appropriate—skipping or hopping offer a powerful protective stimulus. A smaller group with high conditioning may progress to advanced drills, adding variety and further challenge.

The overarching message is clear: introduced carefully, progressed thoughtfully, and performed consistently, impact loading becomes a central strategy for preserving bone health during and after cancer treatment.

CHAPTER 12

Cancer Cachexia — Understanding and Countering Catabolic Muscle Loss

Cachexia is one of the most challenging and misunderstood problems in cancer care. Many people notice weight loss, declining strength, a shrinking appetite, or visible muscle wasting during treatment, and assume they are simply "not eating enough" or "getting out of shape." But cancer cachexia is not ordinary weight loss, and it is not caused by lack of effort. It is a distinct metabolic syndrome driven by cancer biology, treatments, inflammation, and changes in how the body uses energy and protein.

Cachexia affects a large proportion of people with advanced cancer and contributes significantly to weakness, fatigue, reduced treatment tolerance, poor function, and lower survival. Yet it is rarely explained clearly, which leaves many people feeling confused, frightened, or even blamed for changes that are entirely biological.

In this chapter, I explain what cachexia is, why it happens, and how exercise, especially resistance training, can help slow, stabilize, and sometimes reverse its effects when combined with appropriate nutrition and medical care. Understanding the biology gives you back a sense of control. Muscle loss is not inevitable, and exercise remains a powerful therapy even in the most complex situations.

What Cachexia Is — and What It Is Not

Cachexia is a metabolic and inflammatory syndrome that leads to ongoing loss of muscle, and often fat, even when a person is making every effort to eat well. It is not:

- ordinary weight loss
- "getting weaker" from resting too much
- loss of fitness

- malnutrition alone
- a lack of willpower or motivation

Cachexia has three defining features:

Loss of muscle mass. Muscle loss is the central change. Fat loss may also occur, but the primary problem is accelerated breakdown of muscle protein.

Inflammation and metabolic disruption. Cancer cells release signals that alter the way the body handles energy, protein, and appetite. Cytokines such as IL-6 and TNF-alpha increase muscle breakdown and suppress appetite.

Resistance to normal anabolic signals. Even when eating more protein or calories, the body struggles to rebuild muscle because the pathways that normally stimulate growth are dampened. This phenomenon is called anabolic resistance.

This is why "just eat more" does not fix cachexia. Food matters, but nutrition alone cannot overcome the biological drive toward muscle loss.

Stages of Cancer Cachexia

Cachexia develops gradually. Recognizing the stage helps tailor exercise and nutrition.

1. Precachexia

Early, subtle changes such as mild weight loss, slightly reduced appetite, increased fatigue, or small declines in strength. This is the best stage for early intervention.

2. Cachexia

More noticeable changes, including ongoing muscle loss, poor appetite, reduced activity tolerance, significant fatigue, and difficulty maintaining weight despite eating. Exercise and nutrition still make a strong impact here.

3. Refractory cachexia

Seen in advanced disease when weight loss continues despite optimal care and life expectancy is limited. The focus shifts to comfort, independence, and maintaining daily function. Exercise remains valuable but goals and expectations change.

Why Cachexia Happens — The Underlying Biology

Many people feel frustrated by cachexia because they believe it's something they should be able to control. Understanding the mechanisms helps remove that burden. Cachexia develops because cancer alters the body's chemistry, creating a physiological environment that favors breakdown over repair.

The main drivers are:

Increased inflammation. Cancer releases cytokines that stimulate muscle breakdown. This is not a decision or a behavior—biology is driving it.

Increased muscle protein breakdown. Systems responsible for protein turnover, including the ubiquitin–proteasome pathway and autophagy, become overactive.

Reduced muscle protein synthesis. Inflammation and energy imbalance suppress mTORC1 and other growth pathways. This is why eating more protein alone does not restore muscle.

Appetite suppression. Cytokines alter hunger and fullness, change taste and smell, and reduce the desire to eat.

Increased resting energy expenditure. Some cancers raise the body's metabolic rate, meaning more calories are burned at rest.

Mitochondrial dysfunction. The "energy engines" of the cell become less efficient, producing less usable energy and more fatigue.

Hormonal disruption. Changes in testosterone, estrogen, cortisol, insulin, and IGF-1 shift the hormonal environment toward muscle breakdown.

These factors combine to create rapid muscle loss unless the process is interrupted with targeted strategies.

Cachexia vs. Sarcopenia — Why the Difference Matters

Cachexia is often confused with sarcopenia, but they are distinct conditions. Sarcopenia is a gradual loss of muscle mass, strength, and function that develops over time due to a combination of aging, reduced physical activity, low protein intake, hormonal changes, illness, medication effects, or periods of bed rest. It is common in older adults but can occur at any age when mechanical loading is low. Importantly, sarcopenia responds very well to resistance training, adequate protein, and structured exercise programs.

Cachexia, in contrast:

- develops quickly
- occurs even with adequate eating
- is driven by inflammation and metabolic abnormalities
- is strongly linked to the biology of cancer and the treatments

Many people with cancer have both sarcopenia and cachexia, which accelerates muscle loss. Treatment must therefore combine nutrition, resistance training, and medical management.

The Goals of Exercise in Cachexia

The aim of exercise in cachexia is not bodybuilding or pushing through exhaustion. The goals are practical and achievable when exercise is prescribed carefully:

- slow or stabilize muscle loss
- restore functional strength where possible
- maintain independence
- improve treatment tolerance
- reduce fatigue
- improve insulin sensitivity and metabolic control
- strengthen mood, confidence, and resilience
- maintain the ability to perform daily tasks

These goals are meaningful and realistic. They require precision, not perfection.

Why Exercise Helps — Even When Eating More Is Not Enough

Exercise, especially resistance training, is the only intervention that directly activates the muscle-building pathways suppressed in cachexia. It cannot "cure" cachexia, but it can interrupt the downward spiral and provide counter-signals that slow or partially reverse decline.

The key mechanisms include:

Mechanical tension. Resistance training activates mTORC1 and stimulates muscle protein synthesis, even in the presence of anabolic resistance.

Improved insulin sensitivity. Exercise helps muscle absorb glucose, reducing metabolic stress and inflammation.

Reduced systemic inflammation. Regular training lowers inflammatory cytokines and increases beneficial myokines.

Strengthening of neural pathways. Even as muscle size decreases, the nervous system can become more efficient at effectively activating that muscle, improving functional strength.

Improved mitochondrial efficiency. Exercise increases mitochondrial number and quality, improving energy production.

Improved appetite and digestion. Movement can help restore hunger signals and support gut function.

Better mood and motivation. Exercise supports psychological resilience, which is crucial in managing cachexia.

Why Resistance Training Is the Priority

In cachexia, the fundamental issue is loss of muscle, not lack of cardiovascular fitness. Aerobic exercise remains important, but it must be used carefully so it does not worsen energy deficits. Resistance training should be the primary therapeutic stimulus.

Aerobic exercise must be prescribed with care in cachexia. Long or continuous light-to-moderate aerobic sessions increase total energy expenditure and can deepen the energy deficit that drives ongoing muscle loss. This does not mean aerobic exercise should be avoided entirely, but its volume and frequency require careful control. Short, symptom-guided sessions — often accumulated in small bouts across the day — are usually best. If the muscle loss is severe and rapid then light to moderate aerobic exercise should be totally excluded.

High-intensity interval training (HIIT), when tolerated, offers a useful alternative because it improves mitochondrial efficiency with minimal total energy demand. HIIT sessions in cachexia are short, closely monitored, and kept at a moderate—not maximal—effort. These strategies preserve the cardiometabolic benefits of aerobic exercise without compromising the anabolic stimulus needed to protect muscle.

A helpful model for structuring exercise is:

Resistance training as the primary therapy.

Two to three sessions per week, focusing on multi-joint exercises, using loads that bring muscles close to fatigue with longer rests to allow recovery.

Aerobic exercise as supplemental therapy.

Short to moderate sessions such as walking, cycling, or light intervals.

Avoid high-volume steady-state training.

Schedule aerobic work on alternate days or well away from strength sessions.

Exercise on difficult weeks.

On "amber" or "red" days, very light sessions help maintain movement and confidence without draining recovery capacity.

How to Train Safely and Effectively in Cachexia

Training in cachexia follows specific principles to maximize benefit and minimize risk.

- Train close to fatigue, not into exhaustion.
- Aim to finish each set with one to three good repetitions in reserve. Technique always comes first.
- Use longer rest periods.
- Cachexia reduces the body's ability to recover between sets. Rest two to three minutes when needed.
- Limit aerobic exercise volume. Ten to twenty minutes of gentle to moderate aerobic work is usually enough unless advised otherwise.
- Eat protein soon after training. This takes advantage of the period when the muscle is most receptive to repair.
- Autoregulate every session.
- Adjust sets, reps, or load depending on fatigue, appetite, sleep, and treatment effects.
- Focus on functional patterns. Sit-to-stands, step-ups, loaded carries, rows, and presses deliver the greatest return for daily living.
- Avoid high-impact loading. Bones may be fragile. Use controlled, supported patterns.
- Protect energy balance. Training should not increase the energy deficit. Sleep and nutrition are part of the prescription.

Progress in cachexia is monitored differently from other clinical settings. Body weight is not a reliable indicator because fluid shifts, appetite fluctuation, and changes in fat mass can mask underlying muscle loss or gain. Instead, I assess lean mass directly through DEXA scans where available, and I pair this with simple strength and function tests such as grip strength, sit-to-stand performance, or standard strength tests. Stabilizing lean mass is often a major achievement. Even small improvements in strength or endurance usually translate into meaningful gains in independence, confidence, and treatment tolerance.

When to Step Down Training

Training should be reduced when:

- fatigue is severe
- appetite is low
- weight is dropping quickly
- dizziness or instability appear
- hemoglobin is very low
- nausea is significant
- sleep has been poor
- infection or fever is present

On these days, shift to:

- below-MED loads
- very low volume resistance training
- shorter sessions
- mobility work
- breathing and relaxation

Consistency matters more than intensity.

When to Step Up Training

Increase the training dose when:

- energy is stable
- appetite improves
- symptoms ease
- strength sessions feel controlled
- you recover well between sessions

This is how progressive overload works even during cachexia.

When to Seek Medical Review

Immediate review is needed for:

- rapid, unexplained weight loss
- sudden loss of strength
- inability to eat or drink
- severe or persistent nausea
- new or worsening pain

- dehydration
- new shortness of breath
- fever or infection
- confusion or marked fatigue

Exercise is safe when tailored, but cachexia demands close attention to symptoms and clear communication with your care team.

Cachexia and Hope

Cachexia is a challenging condition, but it is not beyond influence. It develops because of biological changes driven by cancer and its treatments, not because of anything you did or did not do. Understanding this distinction helps remove unnecessary self-blame and shifts the focus toward what can be controlled.

Exercise, particularly resistance training, provides one of the most reliable counter-signals to the muscle breakdown seen in cachexia. When tailored appropriately, it supports strength, physical function, treatment tolerance, and overall stability. Combined with nutrition and medical care, it allows many people to slow decline and, in some cases, regain capacity.

The goal is not perfection. It is steady, manageable progress—adjusted to your energy, symptoms, and treatment schedule. With the right plan and support, you can influence the course of this condition and preserve the strength and independence that matter to daily life.

CHAPTER 13

Exercise Medicine for Patients with Metastatic Cancer of the Skeleton

For many years, people with bone metastases were advised to avoid structured exercise. The prevailing fear was that physical activity might trigger a pathological fracture or worsen pain. While these risks exist, avoiding activity entirely leads to rapid deconditioning, loss of strength, reduced mobility, and diminished treatment tolerance. Over the past decade, translational and clinical research has demonstrated that appropriately prescribed exercise is both safe and effective for many people with stable skeletal metastases. When delivered correctly, exercise helps preserve function, independence, and overall wellbeing.

Exercise medicine for metastatic bone disease is now a defined clinical discipline. Research from the Exercise Medicine Research Institute and international collaborators has provided a structured framework that balances the risks of skeletal complications with the equally significant risks of inactivity. The Modular Multi-Modal Exercise Program (M3EP) and the isometric spinal loading approach are key developments in this field. These frameworks enable clinicians to design targeted, safe, and meaningful exercise programs for this population.

Understanding Bone Metastases and Why Exercise Matters

Bone is the most common metastatic site for prostate, breast, and lung cancers. Metastases disrupt the normal balance between bone-resorbing osteoclasts and bone-building osteoblasts. Osteolytic lesions accelerate bone loss, osteoblastic lesions produce dense but brittle bone, and mixed lesions combine both processes. These structural changes weaken the skeleton, increase fracture risk, and often contribute to pain.

Cancer treatments compound these effects. Androgen deprivation, aromatase inhibitors, chemotherapy, corticosteroids, and prolonged inactivity accelerate bone loss, reduce muscle mass, impair balance, and increase falls risk. Without intervention, people can quickly lose mobility, strength, and independence.

Exercise counters these processes through mechanical loading, muscle contraction, improved neuromuscular control, reduced falls risk, and better metabolic health. Preclinical evidence also suggests that controlled loading of metastatic bone can influence tumor–bone interactions, reducing osteolytic signaling and improving local vascularity. Exercise is not a replacement for cancer treatment, but it is a cornerstone of supportive care and a critical strategy for maintaining functional capacity.

The Modular Multi-Modal Exercise Program (M3EP)

The **M3EP** provides a structured, risk-managed approach to exercise in metastatic bone disease. Its strength lies in its modular design: training variables are adjusted to protect lesion-bearing regions while maintaining meaningful stimulus elsewhere.

Core Features

Three supervised sessions per week, approximately one hour each, incorporating resistance training, aerobic conditioning, and mobility work. Progression is incremental—typically 5–10% increases—based on symptoms, performance, and lesion stability.

M3EP Prescription Table

Metastatic Site	Resistance Focus	Aerobic Mode	Flexibility Considerations
Pelvis	Avoid loaded hip flexion/extension; emphasize knee-dominant exercises	Non-weight-bearing (cycle, recumbent ergometer)	Gentle static stretching; avoid loaded pelvic motions
Lumbar spine	Avoid spinal compression, flexion, and rotation	Non-weight-bearing	Avoid trunk flexion/extension; maintain neutral spine

Metastatic Site	Resistance Focus	Aerobic Mode	Flexibility Considerations
Thoracic spine / ribs	Avoid loaded shoulder flexion/abduction; focus on elbow and upper-arm work	Weight-bearing or non-weight-bearing depending on symptoms	Avoid trunk rotation
Proximal femur	Avoid hip loading; emphasize upper body and core	Non-weight-bearing (cycle or arm ergometer)	Upper-limb stretching; avoid hip torque
Multiple regions	Begin with isometric and low-velocity dynamic training	Seated cycle or arm ergometer	Avoid loaded trunk exercise; modify individually

Exercise Modes

Resistance training: 10–12 RM, three sets per exercise, using controlled movement (around two seconds per phase). Train large muscle groups while avoiding direct loading through metastatic sites.

Aerobic training: 20–30 minutes at 60–85% HRmax. The mode is chosen to avoid loading lesion-bearing regions.

Flexibility: Static stretching for 30–60 seconds. Exercises involving spinal flexion, rotation, or compression are excluded when relevant.

Evidence Base

A multicenter RCT in men with bone-metastatic prostate cancer demonstrated improved physical function and leg strength with no skeletal adverse events. This trial confirmed that exercise—when adapted modularly—is safe and beneficial even in advanced disease.

Isometric Spinal Loading for Stable Metastases

Isometric spinal loading extends M3EP by applying controlled axial or paraspinal loading to *stable* vertebral metastases. The rationale arose from preclinical studies showing that low-velocity compression normalizes bone turnover, reduces osteolytic activity, and improves vascularity. Phase I trials in prostate and breast cancer and a phase III trial in prostate cancer confirmed feasibility and safety, with several thousand supervised sessions completed without fractures or neurological events.

Key Parameters

- Suitable for individuals with **stable** spinal lesions confirmed on MRI.
- 3–5 sets of 10–30 seconds at 50–70% maximal voluntary contraction (RPE 6–7).
- Conducted 2–3 times per week under supervision.

Example Exercises

- Prone isometric spinal extension
- Modified supine bridge (hips supported, neutral spine)
- Seated or prone trunk extension isometric on fixed apparatus
- Machine-assisted anti-gravity lumbar extension isometric
- Controlled isometric holds on equipment allowing zero spinal motion

These exercises generate compressive load without vertebral motion, avoiding shear forces while stimulating protective mechanobiological pathways.

Controlled Dynamic Resistance Across Metastatic Sites

With a modular program and isometric conditioning in place, many individuals can progress to **controlled dynamic resistance training**, even when lesions are located in regions traditionally considered high risk. The key is a structured progression that protects lesion-bearing bone while enabling meaningful training of surrounding musculature.

Four Key Strategies for Safe Progression

1. Gradual Load Introduction: Training begins with isometrics and slow, small-range movements. Load increases are small and always guided by symptoms and movement quality.

2. Technique Precision: Alignment is monitored continuously. Exercises avoid end-range spinal positions, uncontrolled eccentric phases, or any action that creates rotational or shear stress through metastatic regions.

3. Autoregulation: Session load adjusts based on daily readiness and pain response. Fatigue, pain, and confidence in movement guide real-time decision-making. Load is increased only when symptoms remain stable.

4. Close Monitoring and Communication: Ongoing communication between the oncology team and exercise professional ensures training safely reflects disease status, treatment cycles, and imaging findings.

Examples of safe dynamic exercises include machine-based leg press, chest press, seated row, supported hip hinge variations, and step-ups adapted to avoid high-risk loading through lesion-bearing structures.

Autoregulation and Pain Monitoring

Autoregulation is central to ensuring safety while maintaining training effectiveness. Pain provides immediate feedback about load tolerance. Mild, stable pain—generally no more than 3 out of 10—is acceptable as long as it does not increase during the set or persist beyond the next day. Pain that sharpens, escalates, or changes in quality indicates the need for modification or cessation of the exercise. Any sudden or focal pain near a metastatic site warrants immediate reassessment.

Daily readiness ratings—capturing fatigue, sleep quality, stiffness, and confidence—help determine the appropriate session intensity. Perceived exertion guides load selection, with most resistance work targeting an RPE of 4–7 while leaving several repetitions "in reserve." Technical precision is prioritized: if movement becomes hesitant or asymmetric, the load is reduced. This approach matches protocols used in spinal loading trials, M3EP studies, and the International Bone Metastases Exercise Working Group recommendations.

How Mechanical Loading Influences Tumor and Bone Biology

Several mechanobiological pathways explain how exercise may affect tumor–bone interactions. Osteocytes exposed to controlled mechanical strain increase osteoprotegerin and reduce RANKL expression, slowing osteoclast-driven bone resorption. Exercise also improves local perfusion and reduces hypoxia, which may enhance immune cell infiltration and reduce pro-metastatic signaling. Muscle-derived myokines released during contraction—including IL-6, SPARC, and irisin—have demonstrated tumor-suppressive effects in preclinical studies. Exercise also modulates systemic factors such as insulin, IGF-1, and chronic inflammation, contributing to a less favorable environment for tumor progression.

These mechanisms are being investigated in ongoing trials using advanced MRI techniques and circulating biomarkers.

Clinical Oversight and Monitoring

Safe exercise prescription for metastatic bone disease requires a structured clinical governance framework:

- Review of imaging (bone scan, MRI) and classification of lesion stability
- Assessment of neurological signs, pain patterns, and functional capacity
- Qualified supervision by oncology-trained exercise professionals
- Pre-session statement by the patient as to level of existing pain and any changes since last exercise session.
- In-session monitoring of RPE, heart rate, pain, and neurological symptoms
- Regular outcome assessments such as 6-minute walk test, chair rise performance, leg-press strength, and quality-of-life measures

- Periodic communication with the oncology team to adapt training around treatment cycles and new clinical information

These steps ensure that exercise is delivered with the same diligence applied to any other clinical intervention.

Digital and Remote Delivery

Digital platforms and remote supervision models have demonstrated feasibility and safety for people with metastatic disease when lesion stability is confirmed. Structured web programs, telehealth, and wearable monitoring allow M3EP principles to be delivered at a distance. This expands access to specialized care and helps maintain continuity during treatment cycles or geographic limitations.

Future Directions

Research priorities include refining skeletal stability risk-stratification tools, determining optimal loading ranges for mechanotherapeutic effects, expanding protocols to osteolytic hematological malignancies such as multiple myeloma, integrating real-time wearable data for remotely supervised autoregulation, and using imaging biomarkers to understand load-driven tumor changes. These efforts aim to create increasingly precise, scalable exercise interventions for people with advanced disease.

Conclusion

The role of exercise in metastatic bone disease has shifted from avoidance to precision-based prescription. With careful screening, modular program design, isometric loading strategies, and close supervision, people with skeletal metastases can engage safely in structured exercise. This approach maintains strength and mobility, supports treatment tolerance, and sustains independence. Emerging evidence suggests that exercise may also influence tumor–bone interactions in meaningful ways. When delivered with expertise and clinical oversight, exercise medicine becomes an integral component of supportive oncology care in the context of metastatic skeletal disease.

CHAPTER 14
Exercise Medicine in the Management of Lymphedema

Lymphedema is one of the most significant long-term effects that can follow cancer treatment. It may develop in the arm, leg, chest wall, groin, or abdomen depending on which lymph nodes are removed or irradiated. The swelling can be uncomfortable, restrictive, and for many people a persistent reminder of their treatment. It affects women after breast and gynecological cancers, and men after prostate, bladder, testicular, or pelvic cancers. Its impact spans physical function, mobility, self-confidence, body image, and quality of life.

For many years, people were advised to restrict activity, avoid lifting, and "protect the limb" by keeping it as still as possible. This advice was based on fear that exercise could worsen swelling. Over time, it became clear that this approach caused far more harm than good—leading to muscle weakness, reduced joint mobility, weight gain, balance difficulties, and substantial reductions in independence.

I started researching cancer related lymphedema more than twenty years ago because I could not rationalize this clinical recommendation given the physiological mechanisms at play.

We now have a very different understanding. Exercise is **safe**, **effective**, and **essential** for managing lymphedema. Structured exercise helps reduce symptoms, enhances lymph flow, improves strength and joint mobility, and supports metabolic health. In practice, exercise often becomes the most empowering and functional component of long-term management. With the right progression and monitoring, lymphedema no longer requires restriction—it requires exercise.

Understanding Lymphedema

The lymphatic system is a network of vessels and nodes responsible for moving excess fluid, regulating immune responses, and maintaining tissue health. Lymph vessels collect interstitial fluid—which contains proteins, immune cells, and waste products—and return it to the bloodstream. Lymph nodes act as filters and immune checkpoints.

When lymph nodes are removed or damaged during surgery or radiotherapy, the capacity of the system to transport lymph is reduced. If lymphatic load (the amount of fluid needing transport) exceeds lymphatic capacity (the ability to clear it), fluid accumulates in the tissues. This is secondary lymphedema.

Early lymphedema involves soft, pitting swelling due to fluid accumulation. Over time, chronic inflammation leads to fibrosis (tissue thickening) and adipose tissue deposition, making the affected area firmer, more fibrotic, and less able to mobilize fluid.

The Impact on Daily Life

Lymphedema affects mobility and function in several ways:

- Heaviness and tightness in the limb
- Reduced range of motion
- Difficulty reaching, lifting, walking, or standing
- Changes in gait and posture
- Fatigue due to increased limb effort
- Greater susceptibility to cellulitis

The skin becomes more vulnerable to cracks, infections, and irritation. Recurrent episodes of cellulitis further damage lymphatic vessels, creating a cycle of worsening swelling.

Confidence is also affected. Clothing fits differently. Exercise becomes cautious. Many people limit activities unnecessarily because of fear or uncertainty—even when exercise would help.

Effective management restores clarity and confidence, reducing fear-driven avoidance.

Why Lymphedema Develops

Lymphedema arises when the lymphatic system can no longer keep pace with fluid production. This is influenced by cancer treatment and several modifiable factors.

Treatment-Related Factors

- **Surgery:** Removal of lymph nodes reduces filtering and pumping capacity.
- **Radiotherapy:** Causes fibrosis, narrowing lymphatic vessels and stiffening surrounding tissue.
- **Scarring:** Alters or obstructs the natural flow pathways.
- **Infection:** Damages vessels and increases inflammation.

But treatment alone does not determine who develops lymphedema. Two major, modifiable contributors—**body weight** and **physical inactivity**—play central roles.

The Role of Body Weight and Adiposity

Being overweight or gaining weight during or after cancer treatment dramatically increases lymphedema risk. This is not a superficial or cosmetic effect—it is deeply physiological.

1. Mechanical pressure from adipose tissue: Excess fat increases limb volume and compresses lymphatic vessels. A larger limb simply requires more lymphatic transport capacity than a smaller one.

2. Chronic inflammation: Adipose tissue secretes inflammatory cytokines. Lymphedema already involves chronic inflammation; more inflammation worsens fibrosis and fluid retention.

3. Impaired lymphatic vessel function: Obesity alters the contractility of lymphangions (contractile segments of lymphatic vessels, each bounded by one-way valves). Lymphatic endothelial cells exposed to high-fat metabolic signaling have reduced ability to propel lymph.

4. Increased fluid load: More tissue volume = more interstitial fluid produced. Even mild lymphatic impairment is magnified in a larger limb.

5. Weight gain after cancer treatment: Research consistently shows: Women who gain **>5–10%** of body weight after breast cancer treatment have significantly higher lymphedema rates. The pattern is similar in prostate and gynecological cancers.

Weight stability is therefore an important part of lymphedema prevention and management.

Sedentary Behavior as a Major Contributor

The lymphatic system relies on movement. It has no central pump; lymph transport depends on:

- rhythmic muscle contractions
- joint mobility
- breathing mechanics
- fascial tension
- posture and positional changes

Prolonged inactivity disrupts all of these.

1. Decreased lymphatic pumping: Muscle contractions create extrinsic pressure that propels lymph forward. Sedentary behavior eliminates this mechanism, causing fluid to stagnate.

2. Reduced joint motion: Joint mobility acts like a natural pump. Reduced exercise stiffens tissues, decreasing these pressure gradients.

3. Muscle weakness: Weak muscles produce smaller intramuscular pressure changes—reducing pump effectiveness.

4. Greater adiposity: Inactivity leads to fat gain, which further impairs lymphatics through inflammation and mechanical pressure.

5. Vicious cycle: Less exercise → more swelling → more fear → less exercise.

In practice, many cases of worsening lymphedema are not related to "overuse" but to **underuse**.

Assessing Lymphedema

Accurate assessment guides treatment and monitors progress.

Bioimpedance Spectroscopy (L-Dex)

Measures extracellular fluid using electrical resistance. It detects very early fluid accumulation before visible swelling. Excellent for baseline and longitudinal monitoring but does not assess fat or fibrosis.

Circumference Measurements

Practical, repeatable, widely used. Measures girth at fixed anatomical points. Good for tracking general size changes but cannot differentiate fluid from chronic fibrosis.

Water Displacement Volumetry

Measures limb volume using displaced water. Highly accurate and widely used in research but impractical for routine clinical care.

3D Imaging and Smartphone LIDAR

Creates precise limb models that capture irregular swelling patterns. Useful for chest wall, groin, and abdominal swelling. Accuracy varies by device, so currently used as an adjunct.

How I Use Assessment in Practice

I look at **trends**, not one-off values. Transient swelling during or immediately after exercise is common and not clinically meaningful. What matters is whether symptoms and swelling settle over the next 24–48 hours. Programs are adjusted based on functional capacity, symptom reports, and objective measurements combined—not one measure alone.

Myths and Misconceptions

Myth: Exercise causes or worsens lymphedema

Modern evidence shows the opposite. Progressive resistance training, including lifting weights, is safe. Aerobic activity is equally safe. In my experience, fear limits activity more than the condition itself.

Myth: Lifting or carrying loads triggers swelling

A properly progressed strength program improves muscle function, posture, and lymphatic pumping. Everyday lifting is safe.

Myth: Repetitive arm or leg movements should be avoided

Swimming, rowing, Pilates, gardening, cycling, and similar activities enhance lymph transport by stimulating rhythmic muscle contractions.

Myth: Heat, sweating, or elevated heart rate during exercise worsens swelling

Normal exercise-induced warmth is not harmful. Increased Gradual progression and hydration are all that is required. Raising your heart rate during exercise does not worsen lymphedema. The lymphatic system does not respond to heart rate in the same way the blood circulation does. Lymph flow depends on muscle contractions, joint movement, and breathing mechanics—not pulse rate. When exercise intensity rises, the muscle pump works more effectively, which actually improves lymphatic return. Studies consistently show that moderate and vigorous exercise do not increase swelling when progressed gradually.

Myth: Compression garments must be worn during exercise

Studies show similar outcomes with or without compression during exercise. The decision should be guided by comfort and individual preference.

Myth: Lymphedema cannot improve

Although chronic, lymphedema is highly modifiable. Exercise, compression, weight management, and skin care can significantly reduce symptoms and improve function.

Myth: Water exercise 'drains lymph' via hydrostatic pressure

Hydrostatic pressure at typical pool depths is modest and evenly distributed. The benefit comes from buoyancy, free movement, and improved muscle activation—not pressure-driven drainage.

The Physiology of Exercise and Lymph Transport

Lymphatic flow depends on both **intrinsic** lymphangion contractions and **extrinsic** skeletal muscle pumping.

Why high-intensity muscle contractions help

Stronger contractions produce greater intramuscular pressure, creating more forceful pumping of lymph. Over time, progressive resistance training improves:

- muscle hypertrophy
- muscle quality (less intramuscular fat)
- capillary density
- mitochondrial efficiency
- neuromuscular recruitment
- strength and endurance

These adaptations improve lymphatic return *outside* exercise sessions as well—during walking, daily tasks, and posture changes.

Water-Based Exercise

Water-based exercise is often recommended for lymphedema, but the reason is frequently misunderstood. Hydrostatic pressure at shoulder-to-waist depth is **not** strong enough to actively "push lymph out." The real benefits come from the exercise environment.

1. Buoyancy reduces load on joints and tissues

People who experience discomfort on land often move more freely in water, enabling fuller range of motion.

2. Greater movement leads to stronger muscle pumping

Water allows larger, smoother, and more sustained motion—precisely the conditions that enhance lymphatic return.

3. Higher-intensity aerobic work is achievable

People can work harder in water with less perceived effort. This improves metabolic health, reduces adiposity, and enhances lymphatic function.

4. Water improves confidence and reduces movement fear

It is easier to attempt new exercises in a supportive environment.

5. Thermal and sensory comfort

Pool environments often feel soothing, reducing guarding and stiffness.

Water exercise is effective because it allows high-volume, comfortable, rhythmic movement—not because water pressure drains lymph.

Compression Garments and Exercise

Compression garments remain one of the foundations of lymphedema care. They apply graded external pressure that reduces excessive fluid filtration and supports tissue stability. During exercise, compression is **optional**. Studies show no consistent advantage or disadvantage to wearing compression during exercise. Comfort, practicality, and symptom response should guide the decision.

What the Research Shows

Across multiple RCTs and systematic reviews:

- Progressive resistance training does **not** worsen swelling
- Heavy resistance training is as safe as light training
- Strength, function, and confidence improve
- No harmful inflammatory responses occur
- Aerobic training improves weight control and metabolic health
- Yoga, Pilates, and water-based exercise are safe and beneficial

- Programs are effective for both upper- and lower-limb lymphedema

Exercise should be part of standard lymphedema management.

Types of Exercise

Resistance training enhances muscle size, quality, and strength—improving the lymphatic pump and function.

Aerobic exercise (walking, cycling, rowing, swimming) improves cardiovascular health and assists with weight management.

Mobility and flexibility exercises restore joint range through scar tissue and swelling.

Breathing and thoracic mobility help lymphatic return through changes in intrathoracic pressure.

Practical Application

People new to resistance training should begin with light loads and progress gradually. The key is monitoring symptoms over the next 24–48 hours rather than immediate post-exercise appearance.

In practice, I monitor heaviness, tightness, and functional movement, adjusting the program accordingly. Most individuals adapt quickly once they realize that exercise does not harm the limb and that transient swelling changes are expected.

Compression garments may be worn during exercise if preferred, but are not essential.

Understanding Transient Swelling After Exercise

It is common for a limb affected by lymphedema to feel temporarily fuller, heavier, or slightly more swollen during or after exercise. These short-lived changes can be unsettling if someone assumes they reflect harm, but they are a normal physiological response. In fact, they occur in almost everyone who exercises; they are simply more noticeable in a limb where lymphatic transport is already slower. The key is understanding **why** these temporary changes occur and what distinguishes expected fluctuations from clinically meaningful deterioration.

Several mechanisms contribute to transient swelling. During exercise, blood flow to active muscles increases substantially to meet metabolic demand. This enhances nutrient and oxygen delivery but also increases hydrostatic pressure within capillaries, leading to a greater—though temporary—movement of plasma fluid into the interstitial space. In a healthy limb, the lymphatic system rapidly clears this excess fluid. In a limb with lymphedema, where drainage pathways are partially compromised, fluid clearance lags behind. As a result, the limb may appear or feel more swollen for a short period.

At the same time, exercise mobilizes interstitial fluid and stagnant lymph that have accumulated in the tissues. Exercise, especially repetitive or rhythmic movement, displaces this fluid and stimulates lymphangion (sections of lymph vessels) contractions. This can redistribute fluid within the limb, creating a temporary sense of shifting or fullness. This sensation reflects **fluid movement**, not fluid accumulation. The system then gradually clears this fluid over the next few hours.

Intrinsic effects within the muscle also contribute. Exercise leads to temporary increases in intracellular water, mild osmotic shifts, and brief increases in vascular permeability—normal consequences of muscle contraction. The muscle belly itself becomes slightly larger immediately after training due to increased fluid content and metabolic by-products. In most people this "muscle pump" is invisible, but in lymphedema it can add momentarily to perceived fullness.

The lymphatic system also shows a short delay in returning to baseline function once exercise stops. During exercise, the muscle pump provides strong extrinsic pressure to propel lymph forward. When exercise ceases, that assistance drops suddenly. If the lymphatic vessels are already impaired, their intrinsic contractions may take time to catch up, creating another brief window where swelling appears slightly increased before clearance resumes.

All of these mechanisms are **normal** and **expected**. They are not a sign of exercise-induced harm, tissue overload, or exacerbation of lymphedema. What matters clinically is the **24–48-hour response**. If the limb returns to its usual baseline within this period, the exercise session was well tolerated and is appropriate to continue. This pattern is a hallmark of normal physiological fluctuation. If swelling remains elevated beyond 48 hours, or heaviness increases session after session, the exercise intensity or volume may need adjusting.

This understanding transforms how people approach exercise. Temporary fullness is not a warning signal; it is a sign that the muscles, lymphatics, and surrounding tissues are responding to increased demand. As conditioning improves—with stronger muscle contractions, improved joint movement, and better cardiorespiratory fitness—these temporary fluctuations often become smaller and clear more quickly. The long-term effect of consistent exercise is **less swelling, better lymphatic transport, stronger muscle pump efficiency, and greater functional confidence**.

The Broader Picture

Exercise works best as part of a comprehensive strategy that includes skin care, compression therapy, weight management, and infection prevention. It restores movement, reduces stagnation, improves tissue health, and supports independence.

People often report improved confidence, autonomy, and well-being once they return to regular activity.

Conclusion

Lymphedema requires long-term management, but not long-term restriction. Exercise is a core component of care. When introduced progressively and tailored to individual needs, it improves lymph flow, mobility, strength, and overall wellbeing. Resistance training, aerobic exercise, water-based programs, mobility work, and breathing practices all have a place. Compression is helpful but not mandatory during exercise.

With structured guidance and consistent practice, most people with lymphedema can safely participate in regular physical activity and maintain a high quality of life.

CHAPTER 15

Exercise Priming – Harnessing the Therapeutic Window

Exercise has an immediate and profound influence on human physiology. Within minutes of starting even a modest aerobic or resistance training session, blood flow increases, immune cells mobilize, vessels dilate, oxygen delivery improves, metabolic flexibility shifts, hormonal and inflammatory pathways begin to recalibrate. These effects are powerful, yet transient, and they occur in the same time-frame in which many cancer treatments are delivered. When exercise is deliberately timed around therapy, its acute biological effects can be harnessed to enhance treatment delivery, increase tumor vulnerability, reduce side effects, and accelerate recovery. This strategic alignment is what I refer to as **exercise priming**, and it functions within a definable **therapeutic window**.

Exercise priming occurs across three phases:

- **Pre-treatment**, where exercise prepares the body and tumor microenvironment.
- **During treatment**, where exercise sustains the biological benefits.
- **After treatment**, where exercise supports recovery, clearance, and adaptation.

Although each phase functions differently, they form a continuum that can turn exercise into a meaningful physiological adjunct to cancer therapy. Some clinicians refer to this as the "exercise sandwich," but the underlying concept is more precise than the metaphor suggests: it is the intentional use of timed, monitored and calibrated exercise to create a more treatment-responsive internal environment.

Pre-Priming Exercise: Preparing the Internal Environment for Therapy

When exercise is performed shortly before a treatment session, it induces a cascade of physiological changes that significantly influence how therapies interact with both tumor and healthy tissues. These changes emerge rapidly during exercise and persist for 30 to 60 minutes afterward, which is exactly when many patients are receiving infusions, radiotherapy, or oral agents.

One of the most important effects of pre-exercise is the improvement in blood flow. Exercise increases cardiac output and redistributes blood toward active tissues, temporarily enhancing circulation throughout the body, including tumors. Tumor vasculature is often disorganized, with chaotic branching, compressed vessels, and regions of low perfusion. These poorly perfused zones receive less chemotherapy, less immunotherapy infiltration, and less oxygen during radiotherapy. A short bout of exercise can increase perfusion sufficiently, in some cases up to 900%, to deliver more uniform treatment exposure. In radiotherapy, this perfusion-driven increase in oxygen tension is particularly valuable, because oxygen stabilizes the DNA damage caused by radiation. When tumors are oxygen-poor, radiation is less effective. Exercise before a radiation session therefore creates a brief period of enhanced radiosensitivity.

The increase in circulation also changes the mechanical forces acting on blood vessels. Blood moving more rapidly along vessel walls produces a dragging force known as **shear stress**, which signals endothelial cells to release nitric oxide. Nitric oxide relaxes and widens blood vessels, further improving blood flow. This widening occurs not only in healthy tissue but also within the abnormal vessels of the tumor, reducing areas of hypoxia and increasing exposure to drugs and immune cells. Greater perfusion and oxygenation create conditions more hostile to cancer cells at the very moment treatment is being delivered.

Exercise also influences the immune system in ways relevant to treatment response. Within minutes, the body mobilizes large numbers of natural killer (NK) cells, cytotoxic T cells, monocytes, and dendritic cells into the bloodstream. These are the immune cells most capable of recognizing and attacking cancer cells, and they play critical roles in the mechanisms of immunotherapy. The surge is driven by catecholamines — adrenaline and noradrenaline — released during exercise. Once circulating, these activated immune cells move into tissues, including tumors. Pre-treatment exercise therefore increases the number and activity of immune cells available to participate in treatment-induced tumor killing.

A related effect arises from the release of muscle-derived signaling molecules known as **myokines**. These include IL-6 in its anti-inflammatory exercise-induced form, IL-15, irisin, and SPARC. These molecules help regulate inflammation, support immune activation, enhance glucose uptake, and increase metabolic stress on cancer cells. The combined hormonal, immune, and metabolic environment is more conducive to treatment efficacy than the resting state.

Another important effect of pre-exercise is metabolic conditioning. Many cancer treatments work less effectively in the presence of hyperglycemia, insulin resistance, or dysregulated metabolism. Even one session of exercise increases insulin sensitivity, improves glucose uptake in muscle, and stabilizes metabolic fluctuations. This more controlled metabolic environment can improve the predictability and effectiveness of systemic therapies.

Finally, exercise performed before treatment has psychological and autonomic benefits. Patients often describe arriving at treatment feeling calmer, clearer, and more physically ready when they have moved beforehand. From a physiological perspective, pre-exercise regulates the autonomic nervous system, stabilizes blood pressure, and reduces the anxious sympathetic activation that can exacerbate nausea or infusion reactions.

A typical pre-priming session involves 10 to 40 minutes (ideally at least 20 minutes) of moderate aerobic activity — brisk walking, stationary cycling, or step-ups — with a gradual warm-up. The activity can be continuous or intervals of work and recovery (e.g. HIIT). The goal is not super high intensity but circulation, oxygenation, and immune activation. Hydration is important, as is avoiding exhaustion. The timing is key: finishing exercise within the hour before treatment takes advantage of the biological window when these effects are strongest, however, **the shorter the delay between finishing the exercise priming and commencing the therapy the better.**

Intra-Treatment Exercise: Sustaining the Therapeutic Window

Exercise performed during treatment applies to infusion-based systemic therapies such as chemotherapy, immunotherapy, targeted therapies, hormonal infusions, or radionuclide therapies. It does not apply during the delivery of a radiation beam. During infusion, tailored exercise helps maintain the optimal physiological conditions created during pre-priming.

Blood flow naturally slows when we sit still for long periods, especially in the legs and arms. Light exercise — even simple ankle pumps, marching in place, resistance exercises, or pedaling on a compact cycle — prevents blood pooling and maintains steady circulation. This helps distribute the infused drug or therapeutic isotope more evenly throughout the body, reducing uneven peaks and valleys that can worsen side effects or limit drug penetration.

Improved circulation also supports oxygen delivery, which is relevant not only to radiotherapy but also to oxidative chemotherapeutic agents. Even light exercise increases oxygen availability and stabilizes metabolic functions during infusion. These subtle changes can reduce the sudden drops in autonomic tone that contribute to nausea, dizziness, and the sense of "crashing" during long infusions.

Muscle contractions also provide mechanical assistance to the venous and lymphatic systems. This "dynamic vascular pump" helps move fluid through the vessels, reducing stagnation and supporting lymphatic clearance. This is especially important for reducing the chances of infusion-related swelling or limb heaviness. Resistance exercises have a greater benefit here but aerobic exercise is still effective.

Exercise during treatment also influences toxicity by improving hepatic and renal perfusion. These organs are responsible for metabolizing and clearing chemotherapy and other systemic agents. When their blood flow improves, drug clearance becomes more efficient, reducing the accumulation of circulating metabolites that contribute to side effects such as fogginess, nausea, and malaise.

I often see patients report less anxiety and better tolerance of infusion when they are allowed to move. Exercise can stabilize autonomic function, reduce sensory discomfort, and shift the experience from passive to active participation. Feeling engaged during treatment can make a meaningful difference in overall wellbeing.

Intra-treatment exercise does not need to be long or intense. Even ten to fifteen minutes can be beneficial and this can be spread across the entire treatment phase interspersed with recovery intervals. The key is safe, comfortable, repetitive exercise such as seated cycling, arm ergometry, or simple resistance exercises. The cannulated limb should not bear strain, and exercise should stop immediately if dizziness, flushing, nausea, or discomfort appears. Hydration should be maintained throughout.

Post-Priming Exercise: Supporting Clearance, Recovery, and Adaptation

After treatment, the body enters a biologically active recovery phase — often more dynamic than people realize. This period involves oxidative stress, immune suppression, shifts in glucose metabolism, mitochondrial disruption, autonomic imbalance, and psychological fatigue. Exercise performed after treatment supports recovery from these effects and helps the body return to baseline more quickly.

One of the key roles of exercise after treatment is supporting the clearance of treatment by-products, not the removal of active drug from where it is working. The therapeutic effects of chemotherapy, immunotherapy, and radiopharmaceuticals occur during and immediately after administration, when drugs bind to their targets and immune signaling is activated. Exercise performed after treatment increases liver and kidney blood flow, helping clear metabolites and inflammatory by-products that contribute to fatigue, nausea, and the lingering "toxic" sensation many people feel. This does not reduce treatment effectiveness; it supports recovery and helps the body tolerate ongoing therapy more effectively.

Exercise also supports immune recovery. Many cancer therapies cause a temporary suppression of immune activity, particularly in NK cells and cytotoxic T-cells. Exercise stimulates immune rebound, improving NK cytotoxicity, enhancing T-cell function, and promoting a more organized redistribution of immune cells. This may help reduce infection risk and improve overall recovery.

Another critical benefit of post-exercise is its influence on inflammation and oxidative stress. Treatments such as chemotherapy and radiation create oxidative injury. Exercise increases antioxidant enzymes such as superoxide dismutase, catalase, and glutathione peroxidase, helping to neutralize free radicals. At the same time, it increases anti-inflammatory cytokines such as IL-10 and reduces pro-inflammatory signals that contribute to symptoms.

Mitochondrial function is another important area. Many treatments impair mitochondrial efficiency, reducing ATP production and contributing to cancer-related fatigue. Exercise stimulates **mitochondrial biogenesis** — the creation of new mitochondria — and enhances oxidative phosphorylation efficiency. Over time, this reduces fatigue and improves endurance.

Exercise also affects the nervous system. Treatment stress can disrupt autonomic balance, increase cortisol, and impair sleep. Exercise helps stabilize the autonomic nervous system, reduce cortisol, and restore normal sleep-wake rhythm. This can reduce nausea, anxiety, brain fog, and the "post-treatment crash" phenomenon.

Peripheral neuropathy is another side effect influenced by exercise. Certain chemotherapy agents damage peripheral nerves by disrupting microvascular perfusion, mitochondrial function, axonal transport, and inflammatory balance. Exercise can mitigate these effects by improving circulation to nerves, reducing inflammatory cytokines, increasing neurotrophic growth factors such as BDNF and GDNF, and enhancing mitochondrial function in neurons. Although exercise may not completely prevent neuropathy, it can reduce its severity and improve functional outcomes.

A post-priming session can range from light to moderate aerobic exercise within hours of treatment. This can then be gradually increased in volume and intensity over the subsequent 72 hours. The intensity and duration should reflect the person's symptoms, energy levels, and safety considerations. Resistance exercise can be incorporated after this 72-hour window as the aim in the initial phase is maximizing the mechanisms explained above and this is best achieved through aerobic exercise. The goal is not to "work hard," but to promote recovery, stabilize physiology, and rebuild function.

Integrating the Three Phases: The Therapeutic Window

Together, pre-, intra-, and post-treatment exercise create a connected biological sequence that enhances treatment precision while reducing toxicity. Pre-exercise improves perfusion, oxygenation, immune activation, and metabolic readiness. Intra-treatment exercise sustains circulation and reduces toxicity during infusion. Post-treatment exercise supports clearance, immune recovery, inflammation control, mitochondrial repair, and psychological restoration.

These effects are not merely additive; they reinforce one another in a way that creates a continuous physiological support system from before treatment to several days afterward. It is this integrated window — this alignment of exercise with treatment timing — that defines exercise priming as a meaningful component of modern cancer care.

Phase	Timing	Mechanistic Focus	Main Benefits
Pre-Priming	0–60 min before therapy	Perfusion, oxygenation, immune mobilization	Improved treatment delivery & tumor sensitivity
Intra-Treatment	During therapy	Sustained circulation, reduced toxicity	Improved tolerance & drug distribution
Post-Priming	0–72 h after therapy	Clearance, recovery, adaptation	Reduced side effects & enhanced recovery

This table summarizes a detailed set of biological processes, but the narrative above shows how each phase works in practice.

Practical Considerations

In practice, exercise priming does not require intensity. It requires timing, consistency, and safe progression. It is more important to stay within an optimal metabolic window. In practice I use wearable sensors such as smart watches to monitor heart rate, breathing pattern, oxygen saturation, skin temperature, and movement patterns combined with patient's rating of perceived exertion. These parameters are combined within an algorithm developed by FitMed (www.fitmed.com) to provide feedback to the patient so they can adjust their effort and time work and recovery intervals. If available then the platform adjusts workload on the FitMed priming cycle to keep the patient within this optimal metabolic window through all three phases of priming exercise.

At the basic level, even a ten-minute session before treatment can improve perfusion and immune activation. Five minutes of exercise during infusion can sustain circulation. A short walk after treatment can lessen toxicity. The cumulative effect of these small sessions can be substantial.

It is essential that exercise timing and intensity be tailored to the individual's condition, treatment type, blood counts, and symptoms, ideally in consultation with an accredited exercise physiologist and oncologist. Prior assessment of physical fitness and exercise responses is essential for the most accurate tailoring of priming exercise.

A note for your clinician or nurse

Timed exercise is increasingly recognized as a low-cost, mechanism-driven tool that can be integrated into infusion centers and oncology clinics with minimal workflow disruption. Compact cycle ergometers, small step platforms, or structured exercise breaks can be incorporated before, during, and after systemic therapy. As evidence grows, exercise priming should be considered alongside established supportive care strategies.

Summary Concept

Exercise performed before, during, and after treatment acts as a **biological amplifier**. It improves treatment delivery, enhances tumor susceptibility, reduces toxicity, and accelerates recovery. This is exercise medicine applied with precision — timed, mechanism-driven, and clinically integrated.

CHAPTER 16

Precision Exercise Oncology: The Clinical Discipline

When I use the term precision exercise oncology, I am not dressing exercise in fashionable language; I am describing a clinical discipline. It is the deliberate use of exercise as a targeted therapy, designed, dosed, and delivered with the same care, accuracy, and individualization as a chemotherapy protocol or radiation plan.

In this discipline, every prescription begins with understanding the person in depth: the biology and stage of their cancer; the treatments they are receiving or will receive; their medical history and comorbidities; their physical capacity, symptoms, and psychological state. Precision means the program is not generic or improvised. It is designed and adapted as a dynamic form of medicine.

The goal is not simply "fitness." The goal is measurable clinical benefit: maintaining muscle and bone despite catabolic therapies; improving cardiorespiratory fitness (a strong predictor of survival); reducing fatigue and pain; stabilizing mood and sleep; and enhancing tolerance and effectiveness of medical treatments. It is also about creating an internal environment that is less permissive to cancer progression and more resilient to the demands of therapy and daily life.

Exercise medicine becomes precision exercise oncology when it is prescribed with the same seriousness as any other first-line therapy. The art and science are to understand who is in front of us, to deliver the right exercise at the right dose and at the right time, and then to adjust continuously as the person and their treatment evolve.

Why Precision Is Necessary

Cancer is not one disease; it is hundreds of biologically distinct conditions. Even within the same diagnosis, individual tumors differ in genetics, metabolism, and micro-environment. Treatments also vary—chemotherapy, radiation, targeted drugs, immunotherapy, hormone suppression, theranostics—each with its own pattern of benefits and side-effects. No two people enter this process with the same baseline health, physiology, or life context.

This is why broad public-health guidelines, while helpful for prevention and survivorship, are never sufficient for someone in active cancer care. At this point, exercise must function as personalized medicine.

A person beginning adjuvant chemotherapy for breast cancer needs a very different plan from someone on androgen-deprivation therapy for metastatic prostate cancer. Their tumor biology, systemic therapy profiles, cardiovascular risk, symptom patterns, and psychological stresses are markedly different. Precision ensures both are treated safely and effectively, with clear clinical intent.

The principle is straightforward: treat exercise as first-line supportive medicine—prescribed, monitored, and reviewed with standards similar to those used for other therapies. When we do that, exercise shifts from physical activity as lifestyle advice to targeted oncology care.

Precision Across the Cancer Journey

Cancer care is not a single event; it unfolds across phases—diagnosis, active treatment, rehabilitation, survivorship, and sometimes advanced disease and palliation. The purpose and dosing of exercise change at each stage, but the underlying discipline remains the same: assessment, prescription, monitoring, and adaptation.

Diagnosis and Pre-Treatment (Neoadjuvant or Prehabilitation Phase)

The period between diagnosis and first treatment is a genuine window of opportunity. Building strength, aerobic capacity, and confidence before surgery or systemic therapy can reduce complications and accelerate recovery. Neoadjuvant exercise medicine (I really don't like the term *prehabilitation*) has been shown to improve surgical outcomes, shorten hospital stays, preserve independence, and enhance tolerance of upcoming therapies.

During this stage I prioritize:

- Aerobic conditioning to raise cardiorespiratory fitness and oxygen delivery.
- Resistance training to build muscle reserves that buffer treatment-induced catabolism.
- If indicated, improve body composition (muscle and fat composition).
- Reduce systemic inflammation and enhance immune function.
- Mobility and balance work to prepare for possible periods of inactivity or neuropathy.
- Education so the patient understands how exercise will be integrated once treatment begins.

For example, a person preparing for major pelvic surgery who is deconditioned and overweight might complete six to eight weeks of structured strength and interval training. In practice, this often results in smoother operations, fewer postoperative complications, and a faster recovery and return to daily activities.

During Active Treatment (Neoadjuvant and Adjuvant Phases)

Chemotherapy, radiation, hormone therapies, and immune-based treatments impose substantial physiological stress. Historically, this was the phase when patients were told to rest. We now know that well-dosed exercise protects the body and can enhance treatment efficacy. During this phase the exercise medicine is also termed *adjuvant treatment.*

During chemotherapy, exercise counters fatigue, supports immune recovery, and maintains functional capacity. During radiation therapy, priming exercise performed immediately before treatment improves tumor oxygenation, potentially making the radiation more effective. For those on hormone or targeted therapies, resistance training preserves muscle mass, bone density, and metabolic control.

The prescription is individualized around treatment cycles and symptom patterns—progressing when energy allows and pulling back when side-effects peak. Autoregulation, rather than rigid scheduling, governs success. For instance, a woman undergoing adjuvant chemotherapy for breast cancer may perform supervised resistance and interval training three times each week. With appropriate adjustment to cycles and side-effects, fatigue can lessen, neuropathy may stabilize, and full treatment doses are more often maintained.

Rehabilitation and Survivorship

After treatment, many people feel physically diminished and uncertain about their capacity. Rehabilitation through exercise restores strength, endurance, and confidence. At this stage, exercise medicine shifts from primarily protective to genuinely restorative.

It is important to target:

- Resistance training to rebuild muscle and bone, particularly after hormone therapies or extended chemotherapy.
- Aerobic conditioning to protect cardiovascular health, especially following anthracyclines or chest radiation.
- Balance and coordination to prevent falls after neuropathy or prolonged deconditioning.
- Return-to-function goals—walking distances, stair climbing, occupational tasks, or family roles—that translate training into tangible improvements in daily life.

For example, a person recovering from colorectal surgery may combine progressive resistance and aerobic training for several months and regain work capacity. A long-term breast-cancer survivor may maintain a program of regular resistance and aerobic exercise, resolving metabolic syndrome and improving cardiovascular and recurrence-risk profiles.

Advanced Disease and Palliation

Even in advanced or metastatic disease, exercise retains its medical value. The aims change—from rebuilding to maintaining, and from performance targets to comfort, function, and autonomy—but the principles persist. Exercise can reduce fatigue, preserve independence, modulate some types of pain, and support mood and sleep. Emerging evidence is that appropriate exercise increases overall and cancer specific survival through a range of mechanisms already discussed.

A person with bone-metastatic prostate cancer, for example, may engage in supervised, capacity-scaled sessions focused on safe resistance and aerobic training adapted to skeletal burden. Improvements in mobility and reduction in symptom burden are common, even when cure is no longer the goal. Systemic changes driven by exercise create a more cancer suppressing environment potentially slowing the disease progression.

Establishing the Baseline

A precise prescription demands a precise starting point. Before I plan a single line of exercise prescription, I need to understand the individual's medical, physiological, and psychological landscape. In particular their risk profile as detailed in Chapter 3. This baseline is the foundation on which safe and effective therapy is built.

1. Medical and Treatment Review

I begin by reviewing:

- Exercise risk assessment, absolute and relative contraindications, and current physical activity (Chapter 3)
- Cancer type, stage, and sites of disease.
- Surgical history—incisions, drains, ostomies, ports, or PICC lines.
- Current and planned therapies—chemotherapy regimens, radiation therapy plans, hormone or targeted drugs, immunotherapy, and theranostics.
- Comorbidities such as cardiovascular disease, diabetes, arthritis, depression, or osteoporosis.
- Key laboratory anchors—hemoglobin, platelets, neutrophil count, renal and hepatic function.
- Medications that modify exercise responses: beta-blockers (blunting heart rate), insulin or steroids (affecting glycemic

control), anticoagulants (impacting bleeding risk), and psychoactive drugs (affecting fatigue, coordination, or mood).

These details reveal both opportunities and constraints. The exercise plan must complement and never conflict with the medical therapy.

2. Functional and Physiological Assessment

Functional testing defines what the person can safely do today and provides monitoring of progress or regress for feedback to the patient, motivations as well as prescription adjustment. I measure or estimate:

- Aerobic capacity—ideally with cardiopulmonary exercise testing (CPET) to quantify VO_2 max, ventilatory thresholds, and cardiac rhythm. Where CPET is unavailable, validated submaximal protocols or simple tests such as the six-minute walk can provide robust alternatives.
- Muscle strength—using handgrip dynamometry, chair-rise tests, or maximal (1RM) lifts (e.g. chest press, seated row, leg press), or machine measurement (e.g. Biostrength, Voltra)
- Function, balance and coordination—single-leg stance, tandem walking, timed-up-and-go.
- Flexibility and range of motion—particularly after surgery or radiation to the chest, neck, or pelvis.

These results guide exercise selection, progression rate, supervision needs, and safety limits.

3. Body Composition and Bone Health

When feasible I use DEXA scanning, which quantifies lean mass, fat mass, visceral fat, and bone mineral density in a single assessment. Where DEXA is unavailable, bioimpedance or anthropometric (e.g. height, weight, waist and hip circumference) tracking still provide useful trend data.

Muscle and bone are twin indicators of resilience. A fall in lean mass signals catabolic stress or underdosing of resistance work; stable or increasing bone density confirms adequate mechanical loading and informs fracture risk.

4. Symptoms and Patient-Reported Outcomes

Laboratory values and performance tests tell only part of the story. Patient-reported outcomes complete the picture—fatigue, pain, sleep quality, neuropathy, lymphedema, nausea, anxiety, and mood.

Short, validated questionnaires and structured interviews help prioritize which problems exercise should target first and provide a way to track the lived effect of training over time. There is an extensive range of general and cancer specific questionnaires which give considerable insight into patient quality of life and mental health.

Expanded Baseline Domains

Precision exercise oncology integrates traditional assessment with emerging biological and digital technologies. The aim is to understand not just how the body performs externally, but how it functions internally as a complex system.

Some of the domains described below are already part of progressive clinical practice. Others are still primarily used in research but point to where the field is heading.

1. Metabolic and Hormonal Status

Key markers include fasting glucose, HbA1c, insulin, and C-peptide to gauge metabolic flexibility and insulin sensitivity; lipid profile for cardiovascular and metabolic risk; cortisol rhythm and other stress hormones to reflect hypothalamic–pituitary–adrenal (HPA) axis balance and recovery capacity; sex hormones (testosterone, estrogen, DHEA, SHBG) which are critical for anabolic drive, bone health, and mood; and inflammatory markers such as CRP, IL-6, and TNF-α to define background inflammatory tone.

In research settings, mitochondrial efficiency may be inferred from lactate kinetics or mitochondrial DNA copy number. Together, these data shape exercise intensity, volume, and recovery cycles, and help identify when metabolic or endocrine support is required alongside training.

2. Gut Microbiome Composition and Function

Stool-based tests such as 16S rRNA or metagenomic sequencing can assess microbial diversity and abundances of beneficial species including *Faecalibacterium prausnitzii* and *Akkermansia muciniphila*. Crazy names but I am sure the discoverer thought these were excellent at the time. Functional readouts, such as short-chain fatty acids (butyrate, acetate, propionate), indicate anti-inflammatory capacity and immune regulation.

A more diverse microbiome is associated with improved treatment tolerance, enhanced response to some immunotherapies, and lower systemic inflammation. Because exercise and diet are major modulators of microbial health, microbiome data increasingly inform exercise and nutrition strategies—training frequency, intensity, and nutritional timing. At present this remains an emerging area rather than a routine clinical tool. For this reason I have dedicated an entire separate chapter to the gut microbiome.

3. Genetic and Epigenetic Profiling

Germline variants such as BRCA1/2, TP53, and others influence cancer risk and treatment selection. Exercise-relevant polymorphisms (ACE, ACTN3, PGC-1α) may influence adaptation, recovery, and susceptibility to overuse injury or overtraining.

Epigenetic markers—such as DNA methylation "clocks" and selected histone modifications—compare biological age to chronological age, informing expectations about recovery and resilience. Transcriptomic responses (changes in gene expression after exercise) show how training reprograms immunity and metabolism at a cellular level.

These tools are primarily research-facing at present, but the direction is clear: over time, a person's genetic and epigenetic profile will shape exercise dose and modality, not just drug choice. Increasingly you will see these integrated into best practice integrative oncology.

4. Immune System and Cellular Fitness

Baseline immune status is gauged using measures such as white cell count and differential, providing a sense of immune reserve and bone marrow recovery. More detailed profiling using flow cytometry can map NK cells, cytotoxic and regulatory T cells, and myeloid-derived suppressor cells. Functional assays such as NK-cell cytotoxicity and cytokine release patterns reveal how robust the immune system is prior to immunotherapy or intensive exercise.

Exercise has the capacity to strengthen immunity markedly when properly dosed. In fact, exercise is probably the most effective treatment for enhancing immune capacity to fight cancer and facilitate immunotherapies. Baseline immune data allow that benefit to be captured while avoiding excessive or mistimed loads. Ongoing monitoring gives surveillance of cancer treatment effects and exercise medicine effectiveness.

5. Inflammation and Oxidative-Stress Balance

Markers such as c-reactive protein (CRP), erythrocyte sedimentation rate (ESR), and cytokine ratios provide a snapshot of inflammatory tone. Oxidative stress markers, including glutathione peroxidase, superoxide dismutase, and lipid peroxidation indices, reveal redox balance.

These markers guide progression: the aim is to expose the body to a level of oxidative challenge that stimulates protective adaptations without tipping into injury or chronic inflammatory overload.

6. Molecular and Systems Biomarkers — Proteomics, Metabolomics, and Lipidomics

Proteomics, using mass spectrometry, can identify circulating cytokines, enzymes, myokines, and growth factors that change with exercise. Markers such as IL-6 (in its exercise-induced form), SPARC, irisin, myostatin, and follistatin show how muscle communicates with the rest of the body.

Metabolomics captures small molecules such as amino acids, lactate, organic acids, and fuel substrates. Patterns reveal whether metabolism is dominated by glucose, fat, or protein oxidation, and how efficiently energy systems recover after exercise training or other cancer therapy. Persistent metabolic inflexibility may prompt changes in exercise load or nutrition.

Lipidomics examines the composition of circulating lipids and lipoproteins and the balance between inflammatory and resolving lipid mediators. In hormone-sensitive cancers, lipidomic patterns may help track how exercise influences steroid pathways and membrane health.

Although these *omics* tools are not yet part of routine clinical care, they deepen our understanding of how exercise alters the biochemical dialogue between muscle, tumor, and host. Believe me, as we embrace truly integrative oncology these tools will become part of best practice cancer care.

7. Psychological and Circadian Health

Sleep quantity and quality, chronotype, and daily energy patterns inform the optimal time of day to train. Mood, anxiety, motivation, and cognition influence adherence and recovery. Structured routines, appropriate light exposure, and consistent sleep–wake times help stabilize circadian rhythms—systems strongly influenced by exercise and closely linked to immune and metabolic function.

8. Digital and Physiological Phenotyping

Wearables provide continuous data on heart rate, heart-rate variability, oxygen saturation, sleep staging, temperature, and physical activity. Over time, these data form a digital profile of recovery, coping, and resilience. When integrated with clinical and biological information, this enables truly adaptive exercise programming—changing load, timing, and emphasis in response to how the person is actually living, not just how they perform in the clinic.

Evaluating Cancer Treatments and Medications

Each therapy interacts differently with exercise. Understanding these interactions turns generic advice into precise prescription.

Surgery often leaves pain, scar restriction, and deconditioning. Here the focus is on early mobility, breathing drills, and specific resistance training, while respecting wound healing and avoiding load over incisions or drains.

Chemotherapy typically causes anemia, neuropathy, nausea, and fatigue. Exercise aims to preserve muscle and aerobic capacity and to modulate fatigue, but load is modified when hemoglobin or cell counts fall. Mobility and light aerobic work continue when more intense training is temporarily contraindicated.

Radiation may cause local fibrosis, pain, and lymphedema. The priority is to maintain range of motion and use short bouts of aerobic work to reduce fatigue. Impact and stretching over irradiated skin are avoided until healing is adequate.

Immunotherapy often causes fatigue and can provoke autoimmune flares. Regular, moderate-intensity exercise can help modulate immune responses and manage fatigue. Any new cough, rash, diarrhea, or unexplained fever demands immediate clinical review.

Hormone therapies induce muscle loss (sarcopenia), bone loss (osteopenia/osteoporosis), and insulin resistance. Heavy resistance training, impact loading, and aerobic exercise are central in counteracting these effects, but fracture risk must be carefully screened, especially in people with osteopenia/osteoporosis or known bone metastases.

Targeted therapies and theranostics may cause hypertension, nausea, and bone marrow suppression. Controlled aerobic exercise supports vascular health, but training intensity and exposure to public facilities are reduced during periods of marked cytopenia or uncontrolled blood pressure.

Safety Thresholds and Stop-Rules

Safety defines the boundary within which precision can operate. The objective is to generate enough stress to adapt, but never enough to compromise treatment and progress.

Typical physiological thresholds include:

- Hemoglobin below 80 g/L: limit to low intensity aerobic exercise and daily activities.
- Platelets below 20×10^9/L: no resistance training; between 20–50 $\times 10^9$/L: avoid heavy loads and impact.
- Neutrophils below 1.0×10^9/L: avoid public gyms, pools, and crowded spaces.

- Resting heart rate persistently above 120 beats per minute or new arrhythmia: stop training and seek review.
- Fever, chest pain, new breathlessness, bleeding, or unexplained bone pain: stop immediately and seek urgent medical assessment.

Symptom-based stop-rules apply regardless of clinical values: chest pressure or tightness; sudden shortness of breath; dizziness or fainting; sharp or worsening bone pain; new swelling, bruising, or bleeding.

For day-to-day decision-making, a simple traffic-light framework helps patients:

- Green days (reasonable sleep, stable symptoms): follow the planned session.
- Amber days (poorer sleep, mild nausea or soreness): reduce intensity or volume, but still do some exercise.
- Red days (fever, uncontrolled pain, severe fatigue): rest and contact the care team.

In the clinic we use autoregulation and teach patients how to use this at home as well. This involves four questions:

1) How well did you sleep?
2) How is your pain level and has it changed?
3) How resilient or vitality do you feel?
4) Has your health changed since your last exercise session or your medical team advised you of anything?

Based on the responses the exercise session is adapted accordingly.

Behavioral Adherence and Monitoring

Even the most elegant prescription is ineffective if it is not performed. Precision exercise oncology depends as much on behavior and environment as on physiology. My task is not only to design programs but to help people perform them consistently.

Anchoring the Habit

Cancer treatment disrupts routine. To rebuild rhythm, I often anchor exercise to predictable daily events: taking medication, a morning coffee, a lunch break, or a specific TV program. The principle is to repeat the same action at the same time with the same cue until it becomes automatic.

Short bouts are legitimate. Several brief sessions across a day can produce comparable physiological effects to one longer workout. The priority is regular exposure to the stimulus, not perfection.

Motivation and Feedback

Fatigue and low mood can erode motivation. Regular, measurable feedback helps maintain it. Objective indicators—step counts, heart-rate responses, strength progression, DEXA-derived muscle mass—provide evidence of benefit. Subjective feedback—improved energy, better sleep, reduced breathlessness—reminds patients that exercise is influencing how they feel, not just what they can do.

Wearables add another layer. Continuous tracking of heart rate, heart-rate variability, and sleep allows early recognition of disease progression, accumulating treatment toxicities or even exercise medicine underdosing. Patients can learn to interpret these signals and adjust within agreed boundaries. This shared interpretation is often therapeutic in itself.

Behavioral Tools

Useful behavioral strategies include breaking large objectives into smaller weekly targets; setting up accountability through scheduled check-ins; encouraging peer or group training where appropriate; and linking exercise to clearly articulated personal goals such as returning to work, travelling, engaging in hobbies, or maintaining independence.

When exercise aligns with values and identity, adherence is driven less by instruction and more by self-direction.

Integration With the Multidisciplinary Team

Precision exercise oncology is most effective when integrated within the broader oncology team. The goal is to ensure that exercise sits alongside, rather than outside, standard care.

The Collaborative Framework

Within the FitMed model we use a five-pillar workflow:

1. Early referral, ideally at or near diagnosis.
2. Comprehensive baseline assessment.
3. Integrated prescription aligned with treatment plans.
4. Continuous monitoring of physiological and behavioral data.
5. Multidisciplinary review to adjust treatment and exercise together.

This framework converts exercise from occasional recommendation into a documented, actively managed component of care.

Communication Pathways

Shared information systems allow exercise data—session notes, heart-rate zones, symptom trends—to be visible to oncologists and other team members. In turn, exercise professionals receive updates on treatment, laboratory results, imaging, and clinical status that influence safety and program design.

This bidirectional communication prevents contradictory messages, reduces duplication, and ensures that exercise is adjusted in step with evolving treatment.

Coordination With Nutrition and Psychosocial Care

Exercise, nutrition, and psychological care form a core triad. Dietitians align macronutrients and energy intake with training load and treatment tolerance. Psychologists address fear, trauma, body image, motivation, and self-efficacy. Physiotherapists and lymphedema specialists help manage regional limitations and local risk.

The combined message is clear: exercise is part of treatment, not an optional extra.

Education and Culture Change

Embedding exercise in oncology practice requires a shift in clinician mindset. The question "Can my patient exercise?" should become "How do we prescribe exercise safely and effectively?"

As clinicians observe that patients who participate in structured exercise maintain muscle mass, experience less fatigue, and tolerate treatment better, acceptance grows. Centers that integrate exercise into care pathways often see shorter hospital stays, fewer dose reductions or treatment interruptions, and faster functional recovery. The clinical and economic arguments support one another.

Quite often I observe that patients actually drive change and this is highly effective.

Monitoring the Precision Plan

Regular review ensures that exercise remains therapeutic rather than habitual. Key domains and example tools include:

- Aerobic capacity: six-minute walk tests or CPET every 8–12 weeks to adjust intensity zones.
- Strength: repetition-maximum estimates or training-load logs every four weeks to track anabolic response.
- Body composition: DEXA or bioimpedance every 3–6 months to monitor muscle and fat changes. For bone health DEXA every 6-12 months.
- Symptoms and patient-reported outcomes: monthly fatigue, mood, and sleep scales to detect emerging toxicity or distress.
- Biological markers: selected laboratory measures or, where appropriate, omics panels at each treatment block to gauge internal adaptation.

The data are summarized and fed back into multidisciplinary discussions, leading to decisions about whether to progress, maintain, or modify the program. And most importantly, provided and discussed with the patient to help you understand your disease and treatment and be an active participant in your care.

Safety and Recovery Governance

Every precision exercise program includes a structured recovery plan. Sleep, hydration, and nutrition are prescribed with the same intent as training. Recovery sessions—breathing exercises, gentle mobility, light walking, or mindfulness—maintain many benefits of exercise while allowing tissues and systems to repair.

This deliberate alternation between load and restoration is what distinguishes training from strain. These aspects are presented in detail in later chapters.

Future Integration

As outlined later in the book, the next evolution in this field lies in digital health and bioinformatics: continuous physiological and molecular monitoring, AI-assisted dose adjustment, and remote supervision. These technologies will extend precision exercise oncology beyond clinic walls, allowing survivorship and advanced disease care to be supported continuously and remotely. Very exciting times!

Conclusion – A Companion Throughout the Journey

Precision exercise oncology is not a fitness program; it is a frontline component of cancer care. It begins with comprehensive assessment, integrates with medical treatment, and adapts in real time to the individual's biology, treatment course, and life circumstances. It respects both scientific evidence and the lived experience of each person.

When delivered in partnership with the oncology team, exercise becomes a structured therapy that supports cardiovascular health, modulates inflammation, stabilizes metabolism, preserves or rebuilds muscle and bone, and improves quality of life. Precision exercise oncology is carefully planned and applied to reduce the side effects of other cancer treatment and enhance their effectiveness. Across all stages of the journey—from diagnosis to survivorship or advanced disease—

the body retains the capacity to adapt. Precision exercise oncology is about harnessing that capacity with understanding and intent.

That is the essence of the discipline: exercise prescribed and monitored as medicine, grounded in evidence, aligned with oncology, and responsive to the individual patient.

CHAPTER 17

Exercise in Complex and Advanced Cancer

Exercise medicine remains relevant throughout the entire cancer journey, including the stages where disease becomes complex or advanced. Many people reach this point after several rounds of treatment, cumulative side effects, long periods of inactivity, or the onset of metastases. Others arrive with profound fatigue, concerns about safety, or uncertainty about what their body can still manage. Precision exercise oncology must adapt to these realities. The presence of complexity does not diminish the value of exercise — it simply requires a more thoughtful, individualized approach, closer monitoring, and a clear understanding of what matters most to the patient and their loved ones.

Exercise does not stop being medicine in advanced disease. Instead, its purpose shifts. Earlier in the cancer journey it may aim to rebuild strength, capacity, and metabolic health. Later on, the primary goals often become maintaining function, preserving autonomy, minimizing symptoms, and supporting quality of life — possibly even extending survival. The common thread is that exercise remains a clinical tool capable of influencing physical capacity, symptom burden, and overall wellbeing, even when cure is no longer possible.

Cachexia is addressed in detail in the earlier chapter; this chapter now focuses on the broader challenges of complex and advanced cancer. People with advanced cancer often face multiple interacting issues such as fatigue, anemia, neuropathy, bone involvement, and treatment toxicity. Exercise at this stage must be matched carefully to daily symptoms, safety thresholds, and personal goals.

Exercise in Palliation and End-of-Life Care

Palliative care is not the absence of treatment. It is the thoughtful selection of interventions that support comfort, function, and autonomy. Exercise remains valuable at this stage, though the goals and methods evolve.

Purpose of Exercise at This Stage

Exercise in palliation aims to ease stiffness, pain, and discomfort, maintain circulation, support breathing, and preserve the ability to perform essential daily tasks. For some, exercise helps maintain the ability to get to the bathroom independently. For others, it supports the energy needed to sit upright, eat meals, or engage with family. These goals matter greatly to quality of life.

Approach

Exercise during palliation is gentle, short, and guided entirely by symptoms. Sessions may last only one to five minutes but can be performed several times across the day. Seated exercises, bed-based activity, light stretching, and breathing drills are usually central. Where possible, supported walking or standing can help maintain balance and functional ability.

Safety is important. People are often fatigued, anemic, or taking medications that affect blood pressure or alertness. Exercises are prescribed to avoid strain, dizziness, or shortness of breath. Supervision by a clinical exercise physiologist, physiotherapist, or trained caregiver can enhance both safety and confidence.

Coordinating With Symptom Control

Exercise is most effective when aligned with symptom management. Light exercise soon after pain relief often feels more comfortable. Breathing exercises can reduce anxiety and air hunger, particularly for people receiving oxygen therapy. Gentle exercise can also stimulate appetite and improve sleep.

Maintaining Engagement

At this stage, exercise often becomes more about continuity and comfort than progression. Participating in exercise can help maintain a sense of involvement in daily life. The goal is not performance; it is preserving ease and autonomy wherever possible.

Exercise in the palliative phase can offer something that many people value deeply: a sense of control. When so much of life is shaped by nurses and doctors attending, symptoms, and uncertainty, even small episodes of gentle exercise allow a person to influence how their body feels, moves, and responds. Whether it is a few minutes of stretching, seated or bed-based exercises, or a short supported walk, these moments restore a measure of agency. They help people participate actively in their own care, maintain confidence in their physical abilities, and preserve a sense of independence at a time when many other choices feel limited.

Hematologic Cancers and Cellular Therapies (CAR-T Focus)

If you are not undergoing CAR-T therapy, you may skim this section. I include it because it illustrates how exercise can be matched to each step of a very complex treatment pathway. The same principles apply across other advanced hematologic cancers.

Leukemias, lymphomas, and multiple myeloma bring challenges quite different from those seen in solid tumors. People often experience profound fatigue, immune suppression, anemia, bone fragility, metabolic disruption from corticosteroids, and long periods of hospitalization. Treatments such as high-dose chemotherapy, stem-cell transplantation, and CAR-T cell therapy are powerful and often life-saving, but they place significant physiological stress on the body. Exercise remains both feasible and beneficial across all these phases, but its role, timing, and dosage must be carefully adapted to the unique biology of these diseases and their treatments.

CAR-T therapy is an excellent example of how exercise can be integrated into each step of a complex treatment pathway. CAR-T therapy involves several stages: first a patient's T-cells are collected; next the cells are genetically modified and expanded (grown) in the laboratory; then conditioning chemotherapy prepares the patient's immune environment; and finally, the engineered CAR-T cells are reinfused. Each step presents a distinct opportunity for exercise to support immune fitness, metabolic readiness, safety, and functional recovery.

1. Neoadjuvant Exercise Before Cell Harvest (Pre-Leukapheresis Phase)

The weeks before leukapheresis — the procedure used to collect T-cells — provide an important window to improve the physiological "quality" of the immune cells that will later be engineered into CAR-T cells. Exercise during this phase improves cardiorespiratory fitness, preserves muscle and mitochondrial function, reduces inflammation, supports glycemic stability, and improves sleep and autonomic balance. These factors influence T-cell health and metabolic adaptability.

There is increasing scientific rationale that the functional resilience of harvested T-cells matters. T-cells that are metabolically healthier and less fatigued tend to expand more effectively during manufacturing and persist longer after infusion. Regular moderate exercise in the weeks leading up to cell collection may shift the circulating immune-cell profile toward less differentiated, more "youthful" T-cell subsets, which are considered favorable for CAR-T manufacturing.

A typical pre-harvest program includes three to four weekly sessions of combined aerobic and resistance exercise at moderate intensity. This can also be delivered across five or six days with the total exercise dosage spread across smaller daily sessions. At this stage, consistency is more important than intensity. Training is always adjusted for blood counts, infection risk, and day-to-day symptoms.

2. Immediate Pre-Harvest Exercise (24–48 Hours Before T-Cell Collection)

Including the Optimal 30–60 Minute Priming Window

Short-term exercise has acute effects that may directly influence the composition of cells collected during leukapheresis. A single moderate-intensity session can mobilize large numbers of immune cells into circulation — particularly naïve and central-memory T-cells, which are the preferred subpopulations for CAR-T manufacturing. These cells are metabolically flexible, expand readily during ex vivo growth, and may persist longer after infusion.

There are two relevant timeframes:

A. Broad window (24–48 hours before collection) Exercise within the day or two leading up to leukapheresis lowers inflammation, stabilizes glucose patterns, reduces sympathetic activation, and improves sleep — all of which support immune readiness. These effects persist for 24–48 hours and help the immune system function in a more regulated, less inflammatory state.

B. Optimal priming window (finish 30–60 minutes before leukapheresis)
Finishing a moderate exercise session 30–60 minutes before leukapheresis captures peak mobilization, when circulation contains the highest proportion of functionally robust T-cells. This timing mirrors patterns seen in studies of NK-cell mobilization and T-cell trafficking, which peak immediately after exercise.

A priming session is usually 10–30 minutes of gentle to moderate aerobic exercise such as walking or stationary cycling. This should not be high-intensity; the goal is immune mobilization, not fatigue. Hydration and a brief seated recovery period are important before the procedure begins.

3. Exercise During the Bridging Period and Conditioning Chemotherapy

After leukapheresis, patients often receive "bridging therapy" — chemotherapy or targeted agents — while waiting for their engineered CAR-T cells to be manufactured. This period may last from several days to five or more weeks. Exercise during this phase helps counteract fatigue, preserve muscle, support immune recovery between cycles, and protect metabolic stability — all critical for readiness at the time of reinfusion.

Conditioning chemotherapy is given immediately prior to CAR-T infusion to clear space in the immune system for the engineered cells to expand. Conditioning regimens are physiologically demanding and can lead to fatigue, nausea, autonomic instability, and significant reductions in blood counts. Exercise during this phase must be carefully moderated. Very light aerobic activity, controlled breathing practices, and small doses of resistance exercise help maintain circulation, reduce orthostatic dizziness, and minimize deconditioning without overloading the immune system.

Even brief chair-based or bed-based sessions during bridging and conditioning help patients enter reinfusion in better physical condition and reduce early functional decline.

4. Exercise Immediately Before Reinfusion (Day-0 Priming)

On the day of CAR-T reinfusion, exercise again acts as a physiological primer. A brief session of low-to-moderate intensity aerobic exercise can help regulate autonomic tone, improve oxygenation, and reduce anxiety. These effects support a more stable internal environment for reinfusion.

These effects differ from those seen before leukapheresis but still support a steady physiological state. Acute increases in beneficial myokines, improved blood flow, and reduced sympathetic arousal all contribute to comfort during and after the procedure. The session is short — often 5–10 minutes of walking or seated cycling — and strictly guided by symptoms.

5. Exercise During the Critical First 7–30 Days Post-Infusion

The first month after CAR-T therapy carries the highest risk for complications, including cytokine-release syndrome (CRS), immune-effector cell–associated neurotoxicity syndrome (ICANS), severe fatigue, cognitive changes, and rapid functional decline. Exercise during this period must be extremely cautious and responsive to symptoms.

Light exercise maintains circulation, reduces the effects of prolonged bed rest, and stabilizes autonomic balance — factors that may influence comfort and functional outcomes during the CRS-susceptible window. Exercise also assists with glycemic stability, which indirectly affects inflammatory patterns.

Sessions typically involve 5–15 minutes of gentle walking, mobility exercises, stationary cycling, or light resistance work depending on clinical guidance and symptoms. Balance exercises help counteract dizziness, neuropathy, and deconditioning. The goal is safety, confidence, and preservation of function — not progression.

6. Exercise in Long-Term Survivorship After CAR-T Therapy

For those who recover well after the acute post-infusion period, exercise becomes central to rebuilding strength, metabolic health, and resilience. Many survivors experience lingering effects from conditioning chemotherapy, prolonged hospitalization, corticosteroids, or treatment-related fatigue. Exercise helps counteract these effects.

Resistance training helps restore muscle mass and bone density. Aerobic exercise improves cardiovascular function, glycemic control, and energy. Gradual reintroduction of combined aerobic and resistance training is typical, although progression may be slower than in solid-tumor populations. Exercise provides structure, purpose, and a sense of recovery after a demanding treatment course.

Why This Matters for Hematologic Malignancies

Although CAR-T therapy is the most striking example, the principles described above apply broadly to leukemia, lymphoma, and multiple myeloma. These conditions often involve lengthy periods of cytopenia, hospitalization, impaired immunity, and heavy treatment burden. Exercise helps preserve muscle and mitochondrial function, maintain aerobic reserve, stabilize metabolism, support sleep, and reduce deconditioning — all essential to maintaining independence and treatment tolerance.

These diseases also require careful adherence to safety thresholds for platelets, neutrophils, hemoglobin, and infection risk. The goal is always to match exercise to the person's physiological capacity, adjusting daily as needed.

Older and Frail Adults

Age magnifies both the effects of cancer and the effects of treatment. Sarcopenia, osteopenia, balance impairment, and reduced recovery reserve make older adults vulnerable to rapid decline. They also respond exceptionally well to appropriately dosed exercise.

Priorities

The goals include preserving muscle and bone, improving balance and coordination, reducing falls risk, and maintaining cardiovascular health. Strength training is especially important since older adults lose muscle more rapidly but also gain it meaningfully with consistent resistance training.

Approach

Training sessions are often shorter and more frequent — for example, five or six days a week of manageable bouts rather than fewer longer sessions. Functional exercises such as sit-to-stand transitions, step-ups, and light loaded carries directly support daily independence. Strength training at around 60–70 percent of estimated one-repetition maximum is safe with supervision.

Recovery and Nutrition

Older adults require more recovery between intense sessions and benefit from higher protein intake to achieve similar anabolic responses. Hydration, sleep, and symptom tracking are essential components of the program.

Special Considerations in Advanced and Metastatic Disease

Certain clinical situations require specific adjustments, and I cover these in detail in earlier chapters. In advanced disease, the principles remain the same — we simply reduce intensity, shorten sessions, and match exercise to daily symptoms.

Bone Metastases

Exercise is both feasible and beneficial with bone metastases, but it must be modified to reduce load on affected regions. I discuss this comprehensively in **Chapter 12**; here in advanced disease the focus is on maintaining function safely. We avoid high-impact exercise, heavy spinal flexion, or rotation near affected sites. Supported resistance training and low-impact aerobic options are preferred.

Neuropathy

Peripheral neuropathy affects balance and coordination. This is discussed earlier in the book, but in advanced disease we emphasize safety: supported walking, stationary cycling, and simple balance exercises with supervision if needed. Nerve recovery lags behind muscle adaptation, so slow progression is essential. There is solid evidence that risk and severity of neuropathy can be reduced with targeted exercise and this discussed elsewhere in this book.

Lymphedema

As explained in **Chapter 13**, progressive resistance training is safe for lymphedema when loads are increased gradually. In advanced disease, we maintain this principle but adjust session volume and rest periods according to daily energy. Compression garments may improve comfort but are not mandatory during exercise if swelling is stable.

Fatigue and Anemia

Frequent short bouts are more effective than long sessions. Reducing volume (not frequency) helps maintain function without overwhelming energy reserves. The traffic-light system described earlier supports daily decision-making. Even brief sessions contribute to circulation, muscle maintenance, and mood.

Digital Support and Remote Supervision

For people who are house-bound, rural, or immunocompromised, tele-exercise programs provide a safe alternative to in-person sessions. Video-based supervision, wearable devices, and automated alerts allow clinicians to monitor exertion and safety in real time. This technology extends access and helps maintain consistency during treatment and is covered in more detail in later sections.

Respecting Goals and Priorities

Working with people in advanced disease requires clarity and respect for individual goals. Exercise should be aligned with what the person values — maintaining independence, preserving mobility, reducing discomfort, or sustaining the ability to participate in day-to-day activities.

My role is to understand these priorities and design exercise that supports them.

Conclusion — The Boundaries of Possibility

Complex and advanced cancer do not diminish the value of exercise medicine; they reveal its depth. When surgery, radiation, or systemic therapy have reached their limits, exercise remains one of the few active treatments available throughout the entire disease course.

Exercise stabilizes muscle, helps maintain metabolic control, reduces fatigue, and preserves independence. Emerging evidence is that appropriate exercise may increase survival and an extension with better quality of life. The focus shifts from improvement to maintenance, but the clinical impact persists. Small, consistent sessions often slow decline and maintain confidence in physical ability.

The aim is straightforward: to help each person remain as strong, mobile, and comfortable as their circumstances allow. When exercise is prescribed with care and precision, it continues to make a meaningful contribution to wellbeing, supporting medical treatment, daily function, and quality of life at every stage.

CHAPTER 18

Physical and Mental Resilience

Resilience is a term used often in cancer care, yet the experience of it is far more practical than inspirational. It is not a heroic trait or a personality type. It is the capacity to keep participating in life — and in your treatment plan — even when circumstances are difficult. In my clinical work, I see resilience as a combination of physical adaptability, psychological steadiness, and the biological capacity to respond to stress without becoming overwhelmed.

Cancer challenges all these systems at once. Fatigue, treatment side effects, disrupted sleep, pain, uncertainty, and increased demands on time and attention all compete for energy. Under these conditions, even the everyday responsibilities of work, family, and home life can feel heavier than usual. Resilience is not the absence of these pressures. It is the process of navigating them while continuing to take purposeful actions that support your recovery.

What Resilience Looks Like in Practice

In exercise clinics, I often see a pattern that illustrates resilience clearly. A patient may arrive looking fatigued, nauseated, or discouraged after a poor night's sleep or a difficult treatment cycle. They may begin by saying they are unsure whether they can manage their session. The safe option is always available: adjust or reduce the session, or postpone it entirely.

But quite often, they will choose to begin — not with the full program, but with something manageable: a short warm-up on the cycle ergometer or treadmill. After a few minutes, I reassess: "How does that feel? Shall we continue or stop here?" Frequently, the patient will decide to attempt one resistance exercise. After one set, they reassess again. Many times — not always — that one set becomes two, then three, and soon they have completed more of the session than they expected.

This is not willpower in the dramatic sense. It is the practical expression of resilience: starting small, monitoring symptoms, and allowing the body to respond. Once exercise begins, biological systems activate that help reduce discomfort — endorphins, endocannabinoids, improved circulation, reduced muscle tension, and better autonomic balance. These changes often create enough of an internal shift for the patient to continue safely.

Not every session unfolds this way. Some days, the body simply does not tolerate more than a warm-up, stretching, or guided breathing. On those days, completing even a small amount of exercise is still valuable. It maintains routine, protects the exercise habit, and prevents the sense of regression that can occur when fatigue dominates multiple days in a row.

Resilience, in this context, is a series of small adjustments and re-engagements — not a single bold effort.

Exercise as a Builder of Resilience

Exercise does not only rely on resilience; it develops it. The physiology of training mirrors the physiology of coping. Each exercise session introduces a controlled stressor. The body responds by strengthening cardiovascular capacity, improving circulation, enhancing mitochondrial efficiency, regulating hormones, and building or preserving muscle. These adaptations create a system that is more stable and less easily disrupted by fatigue, treatment toxicity, or emotional strain.

Psychologically, exercise reinforces the understanding that fatigue does not automatically mean incapacity. Many patients discover that they can function at a higher level than they initially expect, even on challenging days. This builds confidence and reduces fear-driven avoidance of activity.

On low-energy days, a reduced session is still a training stimulus. On higher-energy days, a more complete session pushes adaptation a little further. Over weeks and months, this variability — managed with awareness rather than frustration — creates durable physical and psychological resilience.

The Mind–Body–Immune Connection

The link between psychological state, immune function, and physical health is now well established. Chronic stress and disrupted mood do not simply affect how we feel; they influence hormones, inflammation, and immune surveillance. Elevated cortisol and adrenaline, when prolonged, impair natural killer cell activity, alter gut microbiota, and reduce the efficiency of T-cell responses — the same responses needed to support treatment effectiveness.

Exercise directly moderates these pathways. Regular training lowers baseline cortisol, stabilizes the daily rhythm of stress hormones, and increases the production of serotonin, dopamine, and endorphins — chemicals associated with calmness, motivation, and emotional steadiness. These changes improve immune regulation and reduce chronic inflammation, both essential in cancer recovery.

Exercise also supports circadian rhythm — the body's internal clock that governs sleep–wake cycles, hormonal patterns, digestion, and immune activity. When exercise is performed consistently, particularly earlier in the day, it reinforces this rhythm. Stable circadian patterns are associated with better sleep, improved mood, and more efficient physiological repair.

These effects together form the basis of psychoneuroimmunology: the study of how thoughts, emotions, nervous-system activity, and immune function interact. While the term may sound technical, the principle is straightforward. When the mind feels settled, the body's repair systems function more effectively. When the body is physically active and metabolically balanced, mood and stress regulation improve. Exercise sits at the center of this two-way relationship.

A Practical Understanding of Resilience

Resilience in cancer care is not a matter of pushing harder or adopting a relentlessly positive outlook. It is the ability to continue taking intentional steps — small or large — toward recovery, even when conditions are imperfect. It is built gradually through consistent activity, appropriate rest, symptom-aware adjustments, and routines that stabilize the body's internal environment.

Exercise supports resilience biologically, psychologically, and behaviorally. It provides structure on difficult days, momentum on better days, and a sense of agency across the entire cancer journey.

In this way, resilience is not something you must possess before you begin exercising. It is something that develops because you exercise — a biological and psychological capacity that grows with practice. It is, quite literally, medicine generated from within.

CHAPTER 19

Sleep as Medicine: Restoring the Body's Overnight Repair System

Sleep is one of the most powerful forms of medicine we have, yet it is also one of the most overlooked. In cancer care it often receives less attention than it deserves. People talk about exercise, nutrition, scans, blood tests, and side effects, but sleep sits quietly in the background performing work that no treatment, tablet, or technique can fully replace. When I support patients through their cancer treatment, I treat sleep as part of their therapy plan. It is not an afterthought or a luxury. It is a biological necessity that helps the body recover, heal, and cope with the many demands that cancer places upon it.

Most people think of sleep as rest. In reality, sleep is an active and carefully coordinated state that affects every major system in the body. During sleep the immune system recalibrates itself, inflammatory markers drop, growth hormone rises, damaged tissues repair, and the brain clears waste products that accumulate during the day. Metabolic health also depends on sleep. Appetite hormones, blood glucose regulation, energy balance, and muscle recovery all respond directly to how well someone sleeps.

For people living with cancer or recovering after treatment, this overnight repair system is more important than at any other time. The body is under stress. Treatments create inflammation, fatigue, hormonal imbalances, and emotional strain. Surgery adds pain and disruption. Radiation affects the local tissue environment and the body's energy systems. Chemotherapy alters metabolism, immunity, digestion, and temperature control. All of these pressures increase the body's need for stable, restorative sleep. At the same time, sleep becomes more fragile and more easily disrupted.

This is why in some ways we can consider sleep to be medicine. You do not need perfect sleep every night for it to be effective. You simply need predictable rhythms, supportive habits, and a plan that helps your body return to a stable pattern even after disrupted nights. In this chapter, I explain how sleep works, why it becomes disrupted during cancer care, and how you can rebuild a strong sleep system by using exercise, nutrition, psychological strategies, and simple environmental adjustments. I also discuss the role of steroids and other treatments, how sleep affects the immune system, and what caregivers can do to protect their own sleep.

Why Sleep Matters So Much in Cancer

Sleep provides the body with one of its strongest opportunities to restore balance. Every night, if the conditions are right, your body enters phases that perform different jobs. Deep sleep supports physical repair, including rebuilding muscle, regulating immune cells, and lowering inflammation. REM sleep supports emotional recovery, memory, mood regulation, and cognitive clarity. Light sleep helps the brain transition smoothly between these states and maintains rhythm stability.

Cancer treatment adds considerable strain to this system. Fatigue becomes more pronounced, yet sleep becomes more unpredictable. People often describe lying awake for hours, waking frequently, or feeling unrefreshed even after a full night in bed. Many assume that this is simply part of the cancer experience and that nothing can be done. However, with the right strategies, sleep can improve dramatically, and when sleep improves, everything else becomes easier, including exercise, appetite, mood, energy, and treatment tolerance.

One of the most compelling reasons sleep matters in cancer is its relationship with immune function. Natural killer cells, T cells, and other immune components perform essential regulatory work during deep sleep. Their ability to identify and respond to abnormal cells improves after consolidated sleep. Even one poor night can weaken their activity, but the impressive fact is how quickly they rebound when sleep improves. This makes sleep a powerful tool for supporting the internal environment the body needs during cancer therapy.

Metabolic health also depends on sleep. Poor sleep increases insulin resistance, affects appetite hormones, and pushes metabolism toward storing fat rather than using it effectively. Many people notice increased cravings, reduced energy for exercise, or more difficulty regulating blood sugar when sleep is compromised. When sleep stabilizes, these challenges become more manageable.

Mood and emotional resilience rely on sleep as well. People who sleep better feel more grounded, more optimistic, and more able to cope with uncertainty. They often describe having a clearer mind, better attention, and a greater sense of control.

Sleep is not optional in cancer care. It is part of your treatment.

How Cancer and Its Treatments Disrupt Sleep

Sleep problems in cancer rarely come from a single cause. Instead, they arise from a combination of physical symptoms, treatment effects, emotional reactions, and changes in daily routine.

Pain is a major contributor. Even mild pain can make it difficult for the nervous system to relax enough to enter deep sleep. Neuropathy causes tingling or burning in the hands or feet that often worsens at night when distractions fade. Stiffness after surgery, muscle cramps, and inflammatory discomfort also interfere with sleep.

Hot flashes and night sweats are common during hormone therapy, chemotherapy, and certain targeted treatments. These episodes can happen several times a night and create a pattern of waking that becomes difficult to break. People sometimes worry about the meaning of these symptoms, which adds another layer of stress.

Digestive changes become more noticeable at night. Nausea, reflux, bloating, or delayed stomach emptying can make lying down uncomfortable. Some people avoid eating in the evening because of nausea or reflux. This can sometimes lead to early-morning waking if overall food intake during the day has been low, as the body becomes more alert when it expects energy. For many people, a small, earlier evening meal followed by a 12–14 hour overnight fast works well and supports circadian rhythm. The key is ensuring that total daytime nutrition is adequate so the overnight fast is comfortable rather than stressful to the system.

Emotional factors are powerful. Anxiety, fear, uncertainty, and hypervigilance are understandable responses to cancer. For many people, these feelings rise in the evening when the day becomes quieter. The mind becomes more active, and thoughts feel more intrusive. This creates a physiological state that is not compatible with sleep. The nervous system stays alert, monitoring for threats, and the body remains in a semi-activated state.

Steroids add further complexity. These medications support treatment effectiveness, reduce inflammation, and prevent nausea, but they also raise alertness and blood glucose. If taken late in the day, they interfere with sleep onset and reduce sleep depth. Patients often describe lying awake feeling wired, even when they feel exhausted.

Daily routines change during treatment. Appointment times may be early in the morning or late in the afternoon. Meals may be irregular. Physical activity may decrease because of fatigue, pain, or uncertainty about what is safe. Sunlight exposure may be limited. Hospital stays break natural rhythms. All these factors weaken the circadian rhythm.

The good news is that each of these challenges can be addressed. You do not have to fix everything at once. Even small improvements in one area can create positive effects in others.

Understanding the Sleep System: Sleep Drive and Circadian Rhythm

Two systems control sleep: the sleep drive and the circadian rhythm. Understanding these helps you target sleep more effectively.

The sleep drive builds steadily across the day. The longer you are awake, the stronger the pressure becomes. Physical activity increases this pressure, which is why exercise is so valuable for sleep.

The circadian rhythm is the internal 24-hour clock that governs when you feel awake or sleepy. It also regulates hormone release, temperature, digestion, and energy levels. Light is the strongest signal for this rhythm. Morning light tells the body it is daytime and helps set the timer for sleep later that night. Exercise, meal timing, social interaction, and temperature also influence the clock.

During cancer treatment, both systems become disrupted. Fatigue may cause daytime napping, which reduces the sleep drive. Reduced movement weakens the circadian signal. Low light exposure interferes with timing cues. Irregular meals confuse the digestive rhythm. Stress hormones alter the body's readiness for sleep.

Rebuilding predictable cues restores order. This does not require strict routines. It simply requires consistency in a few key areas, such as waking around the same time, getting outside in the morning light, moving regularly, and having reasonably steady meal times.

When these rhythms strengthen, sleep becomes easier.

Exercise as a Direct Treatment for Sleep Problems

Exercise is one of the most reliable tools for improving sleep in people with cancer. It works through several interconnected pathways. When you exercise, your body temperature increases. After exercise, temperature gradually falls, signaling the brain that sleep later in the evening will be easier. Exercise also reduces inflammation, stabilizes appetite hormones, improves insulin sensitivity, lowers muscle tension, and reduces anxiety. Each of these changes directly supports sleep.

Different forms of exercise offer different benefits. Aerobic training strengthens the circadian rhythm. Resistance training reduces pain, supports physical function, and enhances metabolic control. Mind body practices such as yoga or tai chi calm the nervous system and can be used effectively in the evening.

Timing matters. Morning or early afternoon exercise anchors the circadian rhythm and provides the strongest sleep benefit. High intensity exercise late at night can delay sleep for some people, but this varies. Many patients tell me that they sleep better on days when they exercise vigorously because they feel more relaxed physically and mentally.

On steroid days, morning exercise becomes especially important. Steroids increase alertness, raise blood glucose, and disrupt sleep pressure. Morning exercise helps use some of that alertness constructively and shifts the body back toward a more normal rhythm.

Exercise does not need to be perfect to help. Consistency matters more than duration or intensity. Even a ten-minute walk can influence sleep positively by reinforcing the rhythm of the day.

On days when fatigue feels overwhelming, I encourage people to move gently rather than become completely inactive. Light stretching, slow walking, or a few minutes of strength or mobility work keeps the sleep system functioning. The goal is to maintain rhythm, not achieve high performance.

Nutrition and Sleep: Creating a Stable Internal Environment

Nutrition strongly influences sleep, yet it is rarely discussed in cancer care. What and when you eat affects hormones, digestion, metabolism, and blood glucose, all of which influence sleep.

A consistent eating pattern helps stabilize the circadian rhythm. Large gaps between meals or irregular eating times confuse the digestive system and create unpredictable energy swings. Having meals at reasonably steady times helps align the rhythm.

Dinner plays a significant role. A balanced evening meal containing protein, vegetables, fiber, and slow digesting carbohydrates supports stable blood glucose overnight. This reduces the risk of waking due to hunger or glucose fluctuations. Heavy, high fat meals close to bedtime may cause discomfort or reflux. Many patients with reflux benefit from eating their evening meal a little earlier and remaining upright for an hour afterward.

Some people benefit from a small snack before bed, especially if appetite is reduced during the day, if treatments increase nighttime hunger, or if steroids shift glucose patterns. A small yogurt, banana, or a few nuts helps stabilize blood sugar without causing digestive discomfort.

Caffeine timing is important. Caffeine remains active in the body for many hours, so avoiding it after midday improves sleep onset. Patients who take steroids should be particularly cautious, as caffeine adds to the stimulating effects.

Alcohol may make people feel sleepy initially, but it fragments sleep, reduces deep sleep, and increases overnight waking. For people undergoing cancer treatment, who already have increased inflammation and metabolic stress, alcohol tends to reduce resilience rather than support it.

Hydration patterns also matter. Drinking enough during the day is important, but reducing fluid intake one to two hours before bed helps minimize nighttime waking with need to urinate.

Foods containing melatonin precursors such as tart cherries, kiwi fruit, oats, dairy, and nuts can offer small benefits but should not be expected to fix sleep problems on their own. They are supportive additions within a broader strategy.

Nutrition and sleep work together in a feedback loop. Improving one often improves the other.

Psychological Strategies for Better Sleep

Sleep is not only physical. It is also a psychological experience. Many people with cancer describe their mind becoming most active at night. Thoughts become louder. Fears feel sharper. The quiet of the night creates space for questions that feel easier to ignore during the day. The nervous system remains activated, and the transition into sleep becomes difficult.

Psychological strategies help calm the mind and ease the passage into sleep. The most effective is a wind down routine. This does not need to be complicated or lengthy. It simply needs to be predictable. A warm shower, gentle stretching, slow breathing, quiet reading, or listening to calm music helps signal that the day is coming to an end. The brain responds to repetition. Over time, this routine becomes a cue for relaxation.

Managing mental load is also essential. Many people try to go to bed with their thoughts still active, planning the next day or worrying about symptoms. Writing things down earlier in the evening helps reduce this mental spillover. A short period of worry time during the day can also be effective. This teaches the brain not to rehearse concerns at bedtime.

Relaxation techniques such as diaphragmatic breathing, mindfulness, or progressive muscle relaxation help quiet the nervous system. Even a few minutes of slow breathing can lower heart rate and encourage calmness.

One of the most important principles is not to chase sleep. Trying to force sleep increases arousal and anxiety. The goal is calmness, not unconsciousness. If you cannot sleep after a reasonable period, getting out of bed and engaging in a quiet, low stimulus activity prevents frustration and reinforces the association between bed and sleep. When sleepiness returns, return to bed. Over time, this strengthens the sleep cycle.

Emotional support also plays a role. Sharing concerns with a trusted person, joining a cancer support group, or speaking with a psychologist can reduce nighttime anxiety. The purpose is not to eliminate fear but to reduce its intensity so that sleep becomes more accessible.

Steroid Timing and Sleep Control

Steroids are essential for many people undergoing chemotherapy, immunotherapy, or certain targeted treatments. They reduce inflammation, control nausea, and support treatment effectiveness. They also increase alertness and raise blood glucose. Taking them earlier in the day, ideally in the morning, reduces nighttime stimulation. Morning exercise helps dissipate some of the alerting effect. Regular mealtimes and avoiding caffeine in the afternoon further stabilize the system. Even with these strategies, sleep may still be lighter on steroid days, but the disruption does not need to accumulate across the treatment cycle.

Managing Common Sleep Challenges in Cancer

Many sleep difficulties follow predictable patterns. Addressing them directly can lead to rapid improvement.

Nighttime pain often makes it difficult for the body to settle. Gentle stretching, slow mobility work, a warm shower, or a heat pack can ease discomfort. When these measures are not enough, appropriate pain relief is entirely reasonable. Using medication to reduce pain so that you can sleep or so that you can move more comfortably is part of good clinical care. Both sleep and exercise rely on a body that is not locked in pain. Managing pain effectively allows you to participate in exercise safely and supports the overnight repair processes that your body depends on.

Neuropathy can be more noticeable at night. Light walking after dinner, stretching the calves, or using a warm footbath can reduce discomfort. Some people find that mindfulness directed toward the sensation helps reduce distress if the symptoms persist.

Reflux and nausea interfere with sleep onset. Eating smaller meals, avoiding lying down immediately after eating, and elevating the head of the bed can help. Some patients benefit from discussing medication timing with their oncology team.

Hot flashes and night sweats are highly disruptive. A cool bedroom, breathable clothing, lightweight bedding, and using a fan can reduce discomfort. Some people keep a glass of cold water nearby or use a cooling pillow.

Frequent waking is very common. Instead of trying to force the body back to sleep, resetting the rhythm by getting out of bed briefly and returning when sleepy reduces frustration. Over time, this improves the sleep pattern.

Sleep and Immune Function

Sleep plays an important role in supporting the immune system. During deep sleep T cells become more active, cytokine balance improves, and natural killer cells strengthen their ability to target abnormal cells. These processes are particularly important in cancer care. Poor sleep increases inflammatory markers and weakens immune responses. Even small improvements in sleep can lead to noticeable changes in how people feel physically and emotionally. Patients often report better mood, reduced pain, and improved exercise tolerance after a few better nights.

Sleep does not need to be perfect to support the immune system. It simply needs to be regular enough to allow these processes to occur consistently. Short term disruptions are normal and not harmful. The goal is to establish patterns that support long term resilience.

Caregiver Sleep: Support for the Supporter

Caregivers play an essential role, yet their own sleep often suffers. They carry emotional responsibility, worry about the patient, manage schedules, and respond to nighttime needs. Over time this leads to exhaustion, irritability, reduced concentration, and physical strain. Many caregivers feel guilty prioritizing their own rest, but doing so is necessary for sustainable care.

Caregivers benefit from the same strategies as patients: regular exercise, balanced nutrition, predictable wind down routines, and psychological strategies to manage mental load. Even small moments of rest help rebuild resilience. Caregivers should be encouraged to ask for support, share responsibilities when possible, and protect their sleep where they can. Their wellbeing directly influences their ability to care.

Bringing Sleep Back Under Your Control

Improving sleep during cancer treatment is not about perfection. It is about creating the best possible environment for the body's natural rhythms to function. Morning light, regular exercise, steady nutrition, and calm psychological transitions form the foundation of stable sleep. These elements work together. When one improves, the others follow.

Sleep supports immune function, enhances recovery, reduces emotional strain, and improves quality of life. It is one of the most powerful forms of medicine available. With deliberate strategies, sleep becomes something you guide and support rather than something left to chance.

CHAPTER 21

Should Exercise Medicine for Cancer Treatment Be Fun?

The idea that exercise prescribed during cancer treatment should always be "fun" is common, and many well-meaning clinicians believe that enjoyment is the key to adherence. Enjoyment certainly helps, and where it occurs naturally it is welcome. But expecting therapeutic exercise to be consistently enjoyable is unrealistic — and more importantly, it misunderstands the nature of exercise as a clinical treatment.

Pleasant physical activity has great value. Walking with friends, swimming outdoors, dancing, or playing golf all support general health, mood, and social connection. These activities are meaningful, and I encourage them. But exercise medicine — the type that produces systemic physiological adaptation — is different.

Activity vs Exercise Medicine

When the intention is to create a therapeutic effect, to influence immune function, modulate inflammatory pathways, support metabolic stability, preserve muscle and bone, and improve treatment tolerance, the required stimulus is often challenging. High-intensity intervals, progressive resistance training, and sustained effort at moderate to vigorous intensities rarely feel "fun" in the moment. They feel like work.

In my own training over the past five decades, I have never regarded a heavy set of squats or deadlifts as enjoyable. These sessions require focus, effort, and tolerating discomfort. The benefit arises from the biological response, not from the experience of pleasure during the set.

This distinction matters because exercise medicine relies on producing specific mechanical and metabolic signals: rapid changes in force, high-threshold muscle fiber recruitment, metabolic stress, and large oscillations in blood flow and oxygen demand. These are the stimuli that trigger myokine release, improve mitochondrial function, suppress inflammation, enhance immune surveillance, and improve the internal environment in which cancer treatments operate.

These adaptations do not occur when exercise is limited to what feels pleasant or comfortable.

The Risk of Reframing Exercise Medicine as Entertainment

When exercise is framed as something that must be enjoyable, clinicians may unintentionally reduce the dose to maintain enjoyment — lowering loads, slowing tempos, shortening sessions, or substituting more entertaining but less potent activities. This improves comfort but dilutes the therapeutic signal.

Golf, dancing, chair yoga, or gentle cycling are valuable forms of activity. They support mood, movement, and cardiovascular health. But they do not consistently generate the intensity, mechanical loading, or metabolic demand required to produce the cellular-level shifts that constitute exercise as medicine.

If we dilute the prescription in pursuit of enjoyment, we risk delivering a sub-therapeutic dose.

Taking Your Medicine

None of this means exercise should be miserable, or that pleasant activities are discouraged. All physical activity contributes to health and well-being. A supportive clinic atmosphere — friendly staff, social connection, uplifting music — enhances the overall experience and reduces anxiety.

But the therapeutic component of an exercise session, especially resistance training and interval work, rarely feels "fun" in the moment. It feels purposeful, demanding, and often uncomfortable. That discomfort is not a flaw in the process; it is a signature of therapeutic intensity.

Like any medical therapy, exercise is prescribed because of its effect, not its entertainment value. Many medications taste bitter. Chemotherapy is unquestionably difficult. Yet the dose is chosen for therapeutic benefit, not enjoyment. Exercise medicine follows the same principle. The environment can be warm and encouraging, but the stimulus must remain effective.

Meaningful Reward vs Fun

After challenging sessions, people often report a profound sense of achievement. The hormonal and neurochemical responses — endorphins, dopamine, improved autonomic balance — lift mood and reduce anxiety. This sense of accomplishment is not "fun" in the shallow sense. It is meaningful satisfaction: the confidence of having done something difficult and clinically valuable.

Over time, this becomes reinforcing. People begin to associate exercise not with fun, but with capability, progress, and control — feelings that are deeply important during cancer treatment.

The Purpose of Exercise Medicine

Exercise medicine is not designed to entertain. It is designed to:

- improve treatment tolerance
- reduce side effects
- preserve muscle, bone, and metabolic health
- support immune function
- reduce recurrence risk
- improve survival
- enhance long-term quality of life

These outcomes require precision, progression, and effort.

Enjoyment is welcome when it arises. But it is not required. And it must never become the organizing principle of a therapeutic prescription.

The goal of exercise medicine is not to create fun — it is to support life.

CHAPTER 20

Enhancing Recovery from Exercise

Recovery is when the real work of exercise is done. Exercise is the signal; recovery is when the adaptation occurs. During recovery, muscle fibers repair and strengthen, the immune system recalibrates, the nervous system consolidates new movement patterns, and energy stores are replenished. For people living with or after cancer, effective recovery also helps reduce treatment-related fatigue, lessens soreness that might otherwise discourage exercise, and lowers the risk of injury or illness.

Recovery should not be seen as exotic treatments or expensive gadgets. At its core it is built on repeatable, low-cost habits: sound sleep, sensible nutrition and hydration, light exercise on the days after training, and routines that calm the mind. Massage, compression garments, or cold-water therapy can be useful for some people some of the time, but they are always secondary to the basics.

A practical hierarchy of recovery

It helps to think of recovery as a hierarchy:

1. Sleep – the body's overnight repair shop.
2. Nutrition and hydration – protein to rebuild, carbohydrate to refuel, fluids and salts to rehydrate.
3. Active recovery and gentle mobility – easy exercise to keep tissues supple and energy flowing.
4. Psychological down-shifting – brief routines that reduce arousal and support rest.
5. Body-care strategies – massage, self-massage or foam rolling, compression.
6. Targeted modalities – cooling therapies, vibration, and other tools. Optional and not essential.

Sleep: the cornerstone

Sleep is the single most powerful recovery tool available. Deep sleep is when repair and growth signals are released, tissues are rebuilt, inflammation is better regulated, and the brain consolidates motor skills and memories.

How much sleep?

Most healthy adults require **seven to nine hours of sleep each night**. For people undergoing cancer treatment or recovering from it, leaning toward the higher end of this range is usually beneficial. Nightly sleep shorter than six hours is consistently associated with poorer recovery, higher fatigue, reduced immune function, and increased risk of chronic health problems.

Sleep is organized into 90-minute cycles of light, deep, and REM sleep. Several cycles are needed for complete recovery. Skipping deep sleep or cutting the night short reduces the effectiveness of the entire process, even if total time in bed seems adequate.

Naps during the day

Fatigue is common in people living with or after cancer, and short naps can be restorative. The evidence supports **short naps of 20–30 minutes**, ideally taken in the **early to mid-afternoon** (before about 3 p.m.). These "power naps" refresh alertness and improve mood without pushing you into the deeper stages of sleep that leave you groggy or interfere with night-time rest.

Longer naps of **60–90 minutes** can occasionally be useful if you are severely sleep-deprived, as they allow a complete sleep cycle including deep sleep. However, longer naps should not be daily practice as they often make it harder to sleep at night.

If you find yourself needing multiple long naps every day, this may be a sign of disrupted night sleep, unmanaged side effects, or another health issue. Discuss this with your oncology team.

Sleep hygiene in cancer care

Certain treatment side effects can make sleep more difficult. Practical strategies can help:

- **Hot flushes and night sweats:** Use breathable cotton bedding, keep the bedroom cool, and layer blankets so they can be removed easily. Avoid spicy food, alcohol, and hot drinks close to bedtime.

- **Nocturia (frequent urination at night):** Limit fluid intake in the final two hours before bed, but ensure you are hydrated earlier in the day. Empty the bladder immediately before sleep. Discuss medications that may exacerbate this with your clinician.

- **Pain or discomfort:** Positioning aids such as pillows between the knees, under the arms, or supporting the back can reduce strain. If pain interrupts sleep regularly, your medical team may be able to adjust medication timing.

- **Anxiety or racing thoughts:** A simple wind-down routine in the hour before bed helps. Dim lights, reduce screens, and use calming practices such as slow breathing, reading, or listening to quiet music.

- **Irregular schedules from treatment appointments:** Try to anchor your wake time, even if bedtime varies. Exposure to natural morning light helps reset circadian rhythm.

The overall aim is **consistency and regular cues**. Going to bed and waking at similar times, using a repeatable pre-sleep routine, and protecting the final hour of the day from stimulating activity creates an environment where the body expects rest.

Nutrition and hydration: rebuild, refuel, rehydrate

After exercise, muscles require protein to rebuild, carbohydrate to restore energy, and fluids and salts to rehydrate. A palm-sized portion of protein at each main meal is practical. A fist-sized serving of carbohydrate soon after training helps restock glycogen. Drink steadily through the day, aiming for pale yellow urine. If sweating heavily, include salty foods or electrolyte drinks.

When appetite is poor, softer foods such as scrambled eggs, smoothies, soups, or yoghurt-based meals are often easier. Dietetic support is invaluable if weight loss or persistent poor intake is an issue.

Active recovery and mobility

Complete rest the day after exercise can leave the body stiffer and more tired. Light activity helps circulation, reduces soreness, and supports mood. A short walk, easy cycle, or gentle mobility session is usually sufficient. Intensity should be low enough to hold a full conversation. Stretching improves flexibility and comfort but does not reliably prevent soreness; keep it gentle and controlled.

Psychological down-shifting: calming the system

Stress hormones and a racing mind prolong the body's alert state. Recovery requires the opposite—rest and repair. Simple, repeatable practices can help.

Mindfulness or relaxation exercises, guided imagery, or progressive muscle relaxation reduce arousal. Breathing methods such as slow diaphragmatic breathing or "box breathing" lower heart rate and support nervous system calm. Morning light exposure strengthens circadian rhythms; dimming lights and reducing screen use in the evening help the body prepare for sleep.

Writing down three small things you are grateful for, reflecting on a positive moment, or sharing a brief supportive conversation before bed can also quiet the mind. These strategies are low-cost, safe, and effective when practiced consistently.

Body-care strategies

Massage, when adapted for cancer care, reduces soreness and anxiety and can improve sleep. Self-massage or foam rolling for a few minutes over tight muscle groups can provide local relief. Compression garments or devices can reduce heavy-leg sensation; for those with or at risk of lymphedema, properly fitted medical-grade compression is essential.

Targeted modalities

Cooling strategies such as cold-water immersion or contrast showers may reduce perceived soreness, especially after endurance work. However, they must be used judiciously. Strong evidence shows that very cold exposure immediately after resistance training can blunt muscle-building signals, and repeated cold therapy may reduce immune adaptation. For these reasons, use cooling therapies only when pain, heat, or prolonged soreness are problematic.

Anti-inflammatory medicines or supplements can also ease discomfort but carry the same risk of dampening natural recovery signals. They should not be used routinely after exercise unless pain is a limiting problem, and only after discussing with your care team.

Vibration therapies, including platforms and handheld massage devices, may offer short-term relief from stiffness but provide only modest benefit overall. They should not be used in anyone with fragile bones, bone metastases, or recent surgery without explicit medical clearance.

Safety considerations

Stop and seek medical advice if you develop fever, chills, new sharp pain, rapidly worsening swelling, unexplained breathlessness, chest pain, or signs of a clot such as one leg that is red, hot, and swollen. Avoid immersing a PICC or central line until cleared by your team. If platelets are very low, avoid deep massage or heavy foam rolling. If you have neuropathy, take care with pressure, temperature, and balance.

Choosing the right tools

The best recovery strategies depend on your goals and medical context. For consistent energy, prioritize sleep, meals with protein and carbohydrate, hydration, and light activity. If muscle building is the priority, avoid cold-water immersion and anti-inflammatories after strength training unless pain demands it. If comfort during treatment is the aim, keep routines simple: gentle exercise, soft protein-rich foods, steady fluids, and calming evening habits.

Sleep and balanced nutrition have the strongest evidence. Light active recovery, relaxation practices, massage, and foam rolling have moderate evidence. Compression, cooling, and vibration offer smaller or mixed benefits, though compression is essential in lymphedema care when prescribed. Stretching supports flexibility and comfort but is not a primary tool for soreness.

The short version

Prioritize sleep. Most people need seven to nine hours each night, leaning toward more during treatment or heavier training. Use short daytime naps (20–30 minutes, before mid-afternoon) to ease fatigue; avoid long naps unless severely sleep-deprived. Support sleep with routines that manage hot flushes, nocturia, pain, or anxiety.

Eat protein and carbohydrate after training and drink enough to rehydrate. Move gently the next day. Use simple routines—breathing, mindfulness, reflection, or supportive connection—to calm the nervous system. Extras such as massage, foam rolling, compression, or cooling can be added if helpful, but remember that cold-water immersion and anti-inflammatories can blunt the very adaptations we are aiming for and should only be used when pain or recovery problems outweigh long-term goals.

Recovery does not have to be complicated or costly. Do the simple things consistently. Over time, these foundations will sustain you through treatment, aid recovery after it, and support your long-term health and resilience.

CHAPTER 22
Non-Exercise Activity Thermogenesis

NEAT—non-exercise activity thermogenesis—is the energy you burn from all the moving you do that is not a planned workout. It includes walking to the kitchen, standing while you prepare food, taking the stairs, pottering in the garden, pushing a trolley, playing with children or pets, bending, reaching, tidying, and even fidgeting. In this chapter I explain why NEAT is a powerful, low-stress lever for fat loss and metabolic health, how to build it into a cancer-friendly routine, and how to do it safely during and after treatment.

The big picture: why NEAT matters

Your body uses energy all day long. Most of that goes to running the basics—breathing, circulating blood, maintaining body temperature, repairing tissue. We call this resting metabolic rate. A smaller portion is the thermic effect of food, or the energy cost of digesting and processing meals. Planned exercise—your walks, rides, gym sessions—adds another slice. Everything else you do, the constant background hum of daily movement, is NEAT.

The reason NEAT matters is that it varies enormously between people of similar size and age. Two people can eat the same food and complete the same workouts yet gain or lose fat at different rates because one of them unconsciously moves and fidgets more. The day's small actions—standing, strolling, shifting posture, light chores—can add up to hundreds of calories. In some individuals the difference exceeds a thousand calories per day. NEAT is the flexible dial that explains a lot of the "why" behind plateaus and progress.

There is another reason to take NEAT seriously. When we deliberately cut calories, the body often saves energy by moving less without us noticing. You sit more, stand less, take fewer spontaneous steps. This adaptive response is one reason weight loss is often slower in real life than simple arithmetic suggests. Knowing this helps. If you are aiming to lose unhealthy fat, you must guard your NEAT so it does not quietly slip.

NEAT and cancer: why it is especially useful

After a cancer diagnosis, many people sit more and move less. Fatigue, pain, appointments, infusions, scans and the understandable wish to rest all play a role. Yet prolonged sitting is linked with worse outcomes for survivors, especially when sitting time exceeds eight hours per day and there is very little intentional activity. The good news is that small, frequent interruptions to sitting—what I often call exercise snacks—help. Breaking up long sitting spells with two or three minutes of easy walking or gentle exercises reduces post-meal rises in blood sugar and insulin. On days when planned training is unrealistic, exercise snacks are the easiest, safest first step to feel better and support weight management.

What "counts" as NEAT

Think of NEAT as all the small pieces of exercise that fill the day when you decide not to be still. Walking with purpose counts—down the corridor, to the mailbox, to the shop or bus stop, around the ward. Standing tasks count—chopping vegetables, folding laundry, brushing teeth on your feet. Household jobs count—dishes, vacuuming, tidying, gardening, watering plants. A single flight of stairs counts if you are safe to do so. Exercise snacks count—two to five minutes between long sits: gentle laps of the room, calf raises at the bench, shoulder rolls and stretches. Fidgeting and posture shifts count—tapping your feet, changing position, a gentle sway while standing. Play counts—ten minutes in the garden with a grandchild or a dog is not "just play"; it is real energy expenditure and it lifts mood.

What does not count as NEAT is your planned workout. That is exercise, and it is still important. NEAT is everything else—the long tail of exercise that keeps your daily energy burn higher without the friction of "getting to the gym."

How much can NEAT help?

You do not need to track every minute to benefit. A feel for the numbers helps you see how small actions add up. Scientists often describe exercise using metabolic equivalents (METs). Sitting quietly is 1 MET. As activities become more demanding, METs rise. Using well-established values for common tasks:

A slow walk of twenty minutes is about 2.5 METs. For a 70 kg person that equates to roughly 60 calories; for a 110 kg person about 95–100 calories. Ten minutes of light chores might be around 3 METs—roughly 35–60 calories depending on body weight. An easy five-minute exercise snack—walking a loop at home—adds 15–25 calories. Five minutes of slow upward stairs is a strong stimulus, often around 8 METs; the numbers add quickly. Light gardening for fifteen minutes sits around 3.5 METs—perhaps 60–100 calories depending on body size. Simply standing instead of sitting uses only a little more energy—on average about nine extra calories per hour—so the real gains come from actually moving, not merely standing still.

Steps can be a useful dial if you use a pedometer or a smartphone. An extra 3,000 steps—about thirty minutes of easy walking for many adults—adds roughly 100–175 calories depending on body weight and speed. The takeaway is simple: a few short bouts scattered through the day can equal or surpass a single short workout without feeling like "exercise."

NEAT and exercise: you do not have to choose

NEAT and intentional exercise complement one another. Structured strength and aerobic sessions deliver targeted benefits—improved cardiorespiratory fitness, preserved muscle mass, reduced fatigue, lower anxiety and depression, better quality of life. NEAT keeps the rest of your day working for you, particularly on days you cannot train. It prevents the "sit all day except for one workout" trap. On a week when chemotherapy leaves you flat, NEAT sustains momentum; on a stronger week, NEAT sits alongside resistance and aerobic sessions to amplify your total daily energy burn.

The sitting problem and exercise snacks

Modern life pushes us to sit—commuting, waiting rooms, screens, paperwork. Cancer care adds its own layers of sitting time. Long, unbroken sitting is the problem; the fix is not a heroic workout but frequent interruptions. A practical rule of thumb is to stand up and move for two to three minutes every thirty minutes you are awake. If that is too much today, do what you can—even one minute helps. Over the course of a day these small snacks act like metabolic tune-ups, resetting the system regularly and reducing the spike-and-crash pattern in energy and glucose control.

Safety first: cancer-specific considerations

Before adding more exercise, check the context. If you are underweight, losing weight without trying, or struggling to maintain intake, fat loss is not your goal. Focus on maintaining weight and preserving strength; talk with your oncology team or a specialist dietitian. There are red flags that warrant tailored advice: bone metastases, very low platelets, severe anemia, unstable heart or lung disease, high fracture or fall risk, open wounds, infection, uncontrolled pain, or recent surgery. In these situations the principle remains "move more, sit less," but the **how** is tailored carefully.

If you have a port or other central line, move freely but avoid tugs on the line and heavy or unfamiliar lifting. If neuropathy or balance is an issue, favor seated or supported NEAT such as seated marching, gentle sit-to-stands with a firm support, or wall push-ups; clear trip hazards. If you live with lymphedema, gradual increases in arm and whole-body activity are generally safe; wear compression if advised and monitor for changes. Progressive resistance training has been shown to be safe for lymphedema risk when introduced slowly and supervised. The principle is start low and progress slowly, paying attention to symptoms and responses.

A two-week NEAT reset you can try

The goal here is to build a habit of moving more without adding stress. The plan acknowledges that energy varies day to day.

In the first week, notice and nudge. Establish your baseline by tracking steps or exercise minutes for three days. Add a gentle increase—perhaps 2,000 extra steps per day or ten minutes of easy exercise after each meal. Set a simple timer for every thirty minutes you are awake; when it chimes, stand and move for two to three minutes. Design your environment to make exercise automatic: place the TV remote across the room; keep a small water glass so you refill more often; store the printer and rubbish bin away from your desk; create a safe "loop" at home or on the ward for one to three minute laps.

In the second week, stack and spread. Keep the hourly exercise snacks. Add two ten-minute bouts of easy walking or equivalent light chores in the morning and afternoon. If safe, add a flight of stairs once or twice a day or choose a gentle hill. Build in play—ten minutes with kids or pets. Check your steps or exercise minutes a few times per day and adjust gently.

Over two weeks, these nudges can add 150–300 calories per day for many adults without feeling like a "program." Your exact number will vary with body size and pace, but the principle is robust: small, frequent exercise adds up.

NEAT menus for different energy days

Energy is not fixed. On a strong day, take a brisk ten-minute walk after each main meal, climb one or two flights of stairs twice, do a fifteen-minute tidy or vacuum, park a little farther from the shop, and make five minutes of kitchen laps while the kettle boils—repeat that short loop three times across the day. On an "okay" day, walk five minutes after two meals, stand and sway or stretch during TV ad breaks, fold laundry or tidy a drawer for ten minutes, walk while on phone calls, and after you visit the bathroom, add two minutes of hallway laps before returning to your chair. On a low-energy day, keep it tiny but keep it going: seated marches and ankle pumps for one to two minutes each hour, a few supported sit-to-stands from a sturdy chair, gentle wall or table push-ups, standing for one minute each hour if safe, and a few long exhales to ease tension before moving again. These are not trivial. They protect the habit loop even when energy is scarce.

NEAT at home, work, and the hospital

At home, place commonly used items—remote, water, phone charger—in another room to create natural walking prompts. Do chore bursts after meals: ten to fifteen minutes of dishes, wiping benches, putting things away. In a two-story home, add a safe up-and-down trip once or twice daily if balance allows.

At work, take "walk and talk" phone calls; if remote, stand for a minute or two each half hour. Place the printer and bin farther away. If a bathroom on another floor is available and safe for you, use the stairs. Put two ten-minute walking blocks in your calendar mid-morning and mid-afternoon.

At the hospital or clinic, ask if there is a safe corridor loop you can stroll for two or three minutes between waits. During infusions—if permitted and you feel steady—perform ankle pumps, gentle foot circles, calf raises or seated marches. Keep trip hazards clear; never move in a way that could pull a port or line. A small loop walked five or six times during a long appointment is meaningful exercise.

Tracking NEAT simply and honestly

Steps are the easiest proxy. A phone, a cheap pedometer, or a watch will suffice. Do not obsess over the numbers; check two or three times per day and adjust. Aim for a steady upward trend—for example, baseline plus 2,000 steps per day for two weeks. If steps are hard to track because neuropathy alters gait or you use mobility aids, track movement minutes or the number of exercise snacks instead.

A realistic note: NEAT supports fat loss only if extra exercise is not fully offset by extra eating. That does not mean you must be hungry. Most people can boost NEAT without triggering strong appetite increases. Simply be mindful of "compensation"—the tendency to reward extra exercise with extra snacks. Spread protein across meals and include higher-fiber foods; both help with satiety while supporting muscle.

Common questions, answered plainly

Is standing at a desk enough? Standing is a little better than sitting—roughly nine extra calories per hour on average across studies—but exercise breaks deliver far bigger benefits for metabolism. The best approach is a sit-stand desk combined with a brief walk every half hour.

Do fidgeting and posture shifts really matter? They do. They are part of NEAT and help explain why some people burn much more energy day to day. Small, frequent adjustments add up across hours.

What if I am exhausted? On low-energy days think in minutes, not sessions. One or two minutes each hour—seated or supported—is acceptable. The goal is to protect the habit without draining your tank. Tomorrow you can do more.

Can NEAT replace workouts? No. NEAT is the foundation; structured strength and aerobic sessions build the walls and roof. Keep building NEAT and add two or three brief strength sessions per week plus walks when you can. That combination is most effective for fatigue, function, and sustainable fat loss.

Will NEAT make me lose muscle? On its own, NEAT does not build muscle, but it will not make you lose it if you pair it with adequate protein and short, regular resistance work. NEAT raises daily energy expenditure; resistance training tells your body to keep muscle. Together, they work well.

NEAT and strength: your fat-loss duo

Fat loss that lasts works best when you protect muscle. Two or three short strength sessions per week—bands, bodyweight, or light weights—combined with daily NEAT keeps overall energy burn higher while signaling muscle to stay. Spread protein across meals and adjust portions slowly. Aim for steady, sustainable change rather than crash diets. Exercise guidelines for cancer survivors support combined aerobic and resistance training to reduce fatigue and improve quality of life; NEAT makes the rest of your day contribute even when workouts are not possible.

A quick NEAT audit you can do today

Take a moment to reflect. Do you regularly sit for more than thirty minutes without a break? Do you average fewer than 5,000 steps per day? Do you have safe, clear space at home for short laps? Can you attach exercise to triggers (phone rings, ads, kettle boils)? Do you have stairs or a small hill you can use safely? Do you have seated options for low-energy days? Do you know your personal red flags and when to seek guidance? Finally, choose three new habits from this chapter to try this week.

Key takeaways

NEAT is the energy you burn from everyday exercise, not workouts. It is a big, flexible lever for fat loss that varies widely from person to person. Dieting can quietly lower NEAT, so plan exercise throughout your day. For cancer survivors, moving more and sitting less is linked with better survival, particularly if you currently sit a lot. Break up long sits with two or three minutes of light walking or gentle exercise; it helps your metabolism. Standing alone adds a little, but short walks and exercise snacks add much more. Build tiny, repeatable habits. NEAT should feel easy—especially during treatment and recovery.

Final word

For many people living with or beyond cancer, NEAT is the simplest, lowest-stress lever for fat loss and better health. You do not need to "work out" to benefit. Move a little more, a little more often. Stand up, take a short stroll, tidy a corner, climb a safe flight, play for five minutes, perform a set of sit-to-stands. These small acts, done most days, add up. Over weeks and months they shift your biology in the right direction—quietly, persistently, and without overwhelming your day.

CHAPTER 23
Diet and Nutrition Therapy

"The type and timing of your eating can vastly impact your weight, level of inflammation, gut microbiome, and even psychological health."

Nutrition: practical food strategies that support exercise medicine

Exercise is the most powerful treatment we can prescribe to build strength, protect function, and lift quality of life during and after cancer. But exercise does not act alone. Nutrition is its daily partner. Food is the fuel that lets exercise do its work; it supports immunity, preserves muscle, steadies energy on long days, and—when the time is right—helps you lose unhealthy fat without sacrificing the strength you are working to rebuild.

I am not a dietitian or nutritionist, and I want to acknowledge that upfront. What I present here is drawn from reading, research, and many discussions with colleagues who are experts in nutrition science. After exercise medicine and mental health strategies, I believe nutritional medicine is one of the most powerful levers for surviving and thriving after a cancer diagnosis.

Why nutrition matters now

Most adults begin their cancer journey with a little more body fat and a little less muscle than they would like. That mix matters. Excess fat and low muscle create an internal environment that is more inflammatory and less resilient. Treatment adds stress; without attention to food and exercise, it is harder to bounce back. Nutrition is how we change that terrain from the inside out.

In practice, food does four jobs. First, protect and rebuild muscle so you can stay independent and strong. Second, when it is safe, reduce excess fat to ease pressure on blood sugar, blood pressure, joints, and sleep. Third, lower background inflammatory tone by favoring a plant-forward pattern. Fourth, work with medicines, not against them—avoiding known food–drug conflicts and using supplements cautiously.

There is a time for everything. During active treatment—especially if weight is falling—the priority is eating enough and protecting muscle. Intentional weight loss can wait. After treatment, or in maintenance phases if your clinicians agree, you can pursue gentle fat loss at a calm pace while protecting lean tissue. The everyday pattern looks similar in both situations.

The outcome we aim for: strong, not just light

The goal is not simply to weigh less; it is to change body composition—more lean tissue, less excessive fat. Strong legs that carry you upstairs, grip strength to open jars, a back that supports you when walking with a grandchild. That is why protein and resistance training are twin pillars in survivorship.

If weight loss is appropriate, aim for 0.25–0.5 kg (½–1 lb) per week. Faster losses almost always strip away muscle along with fat. This is particularly harmful in cancer. Low muscle mass is strongly linked to worse chemotherapy toxicity, more dose reductions and delays, and poorer survival across many cancers. Aggressive dieting pushes the body to break down muscle protein for glucose, leaving you weaker and less resilient.

A slower pace, paired with higher protein (typically 1.2–1.6 g/kg/day) and resistance training two or three days per week, ensures that most of the weight lost is fat, not muscle. It is far better to take six months to lose ten kilograms and keep your muscle than to lose it in ten weeks and end up weaker. Protecting muscle protects independence, treatment tolerance, and long-term health.

The everyday pattern: Mediterranean and plant-forward

Picture your plate: half vegetables and fruit, a quarter protein, a quarter slow-digesting carbohydrate such as beans, lentils, whole grains, or starchy vegetables. Add olive oil, nuts, seeds, or avocado. This Mediterranean-style, plant-forward pattern is flexible and enjoyable. It reduces ultra-processed foods while lifting fiber, vitamins, minerals and phytonutrients the body uses to repair and regulate.

Use the pantry and freezer without guilt. Canned beans, tinned salmon, frozen berries and chopped vegetables are allies. Rinse canned beans to reduce sodium. Keep olive oil, oats, brown rice or quinoa, and a reliable spice blend handy—these basics make good choices easy on hard days.

Processed meats—bacon, ham, sausages, salami—sit at the "occasional" end of the spectrum. If you eat red meat, make it a small side rather than the center of the plate, kept to modest weekly amounts. Alcohol follows the same rule in survivorship: less is best.

Ensuring you get enough protein

Protein is essential for protecting and rebuilding muscle during and after treatment. A practical target for many adults is 1.2–1.6 g/kg/day, rising to ~1.8 g/kg during rebuilding phases if kidney function is healthy. Spread protein across the day; 20–40 grams per meal reliably stimulates muscle growth, with older adults often benefitting from the higher end.

Animal sources include fish (especially oily fish), eggs, yoghurt or cottage cheese, poultry, and lean meats. Plant-based sources include tofu, tempeh, soy milk or yoghurt, edamame, lentils, chickpeas, beans, quinoa, nuts, and seeds. Protein powders—whey or pea—are useful when appetite is low or taste is altered. If you have kidney disease or another specific condition, your team will tailor targets.

Soy foods—such as tofu, tempeh, edamame, soy yoghurt and soy milk—are safe for breast-cancer survivors and most people in survivorship; this reassurance does not extend to high-dose isoflavone supplements.

Inflammation-lowering diets

Systemic inflammation—the low, persistent background hum that drains energy and slows recovery—can be reduced through diet. A colorful, plant-rich pattern with vegetables, legumes, whole grains, nuts, seeds, olive oil, herbs, and spices nudges inflammation down. Diets heavy in ultra-processed foods and processed meats push it up. The principle is simple: meals that look like real ingredients combined are better than meals dominated by packaged, manufactured foods.

Your gut microbiome

The gut hosts trillions of microbes that influence digestion, immunity, inflammation, and mood. Cancer treatments often disrupt this ecosystem. Supporting your microbiome through food is one of the simplest ways to improve resilience.

Prebiotics are fibers and plant compounds we cannot digest but bacteria thrive on. They fuel beneficial microbes which, in turn, produce short-chain fatty acids like butyrate that reduce inflammation, strengthen the gut barrier, and regulate immunity. Good sources include legumes, whole grains, onions, garlic, leeks, asparagus, artichokes, bananas, apples, berries, nuts and seeds. Variety matters; different plants feed different microbes.

Probiotics are live microorganisms. In food, they are found in fermented products such as yoghurt with live cultures, kefir, sauerkraut, kimchi, miso, and tempeh. These are safe and enjoyable ways to support the microbiome for most people. Probiotic supplements are more complex. Routine use in cancer care has not shown consistent benefit and may be unhelpful during immunotherapy. In those with very low immunity there is a rare infection risk. Food-based probiotics are safe for most; if a supplement is considered, do so under guidance from your oncology or dietetics team.

Prebiotics and probiotics work best together. Yoghurt with oats and berries, or miso soup with tofu and vegetables, pairs fuel and friendly bacteria in one meal. In people on immunotherapy, higher dietary fiber has been linked with better responses, while routine probiotic supplementation has not. A target of 20–30 grams of fiber per day, adjusted for tolerance, with a daily fermented food if safe, is a sound approach.

Carbohydrates and fiber: fuel that works with you

Cancer therapy days are often stop-and-go. Carbohydrate is the main fuel for this rhythm. The best sources come packaged with fiber and water—vegetables, fruit, legumes, whole grains. Most adults should aim for 25–38 grams of fiber per day; increase gradually and drink fluids to avoid cramps and bloating.

Fruit is not the enemy. A banana or handful of grapes provides fiber, water, potassium, and protective plant compounds. What we reduce are sugary drinks—soft drinks, sweet teas, juice drinks. Choose water, sparkling water, unsweetened tea or coffee, or milk/soy milk as everyday drinks.

If steroids or other treatments raise blood sugar, the same plate pattern works: vegetables, plant proteins, modest whole grains, and healthy fats. A five- to ten-minute walk after meals helps smooth post-meal blood sugar at any pace you can manage.

Fat quality: more olive oil and omega-3s, fewer processed fats

Fat quality matters. Olive oil, nuts, seeds, and avocado support heart health and fit neatly into a Mediterranean plate. Oily fish such as salmon, sardines and mackerel provide long-chain omega-3s (EPA/DHA). Omega-3 supplements have mixed results in cachexia; when considered, they should be guided by your clinician. For most, including fish a few times per week or adding walnuts, chia and flax is sufficient.

Nutrient timing

Nutrient timing is about matching fuel to need. Start exercise with stable blood glucose—do not begin fasted if you feel light-headed. A small, easily digested carbohydrate snack close to training (fruit, toast with honey) can help if you train early or feel flat.

During most sessions lasting 30–60 minutes, you do not need extra food—water is adequate. After training, combine protein with carbohydrate to support repair and replenish glycogen. The day's pattern matters more than an exact "window"; total daily protein and energy are the priority.

Intermittent and periodic fasting

Intermittent fasting usually means eating within a daily time window (for example, an eight-hour window with sixteen hours fasting). Periodic fasting involves longer spans at very low calorie intake. Large randomized trials in cancer populations are still lacking. Early data suggest fasting is safe for selected people, with minor transient side effects. The rationale is that fasting lowers glucose and insulin-like growth factors that fuel cancer growth and may sensitize tumors to therapy while protecting normal cells.

Intermittent fasting can be a viable approach to weight control. Many people find the "16:8" pattern effective and tolerable. I have used this approach personally: exercise early, eat three substantial meals between breakfast and mid-afternoon, and fast until morning. The meals are satisfying and the benefits for weight control and sleep are clear. The key caveat is that fasting must not compromise protein intake, total calories during treatment, or diet quality. It is not appropriate for people struggling to maintain weight or muscle.

Ketogenic diets have been explored with mixed and inconsistent results, and adherence is difficult. For most, a high-quality, largely plant-based diet using familiar foods is safer and more sustainable.

Eating during treatment: adjust the goal, protect the habit

When treatment is active—especially if weight is falling—the goal is enough calories and enough protein to keep the body resilient. Smooth the path to eating rather than erecting hurdles.

When "nothing sounds good," favor small, frequent meals. Smoothies often go down easier than plates: milk or soy milk, whey or pea protein, banana or berries, and peanut butter. Blended soups are soothing and nutrient-dense. Metallic taste responds to plastic cutlery, tart flavors (lemon, vinegar), and herb-based marinades. Serving meat or fish cold reduces aromas. Many people tolerate eggs, yoghurt, tofu, and beans better than red meat when taste is "off."

For mouth sores, soft and cool foods work best; avoid spicy or acidic foods. For dry mouth, sip fluids often, choose moist foods, and use sugar-free gum or lozenges. For nausea, try plain foods and reduce strong kitchen smells. For diarrhea, rehydrate and temporarily favor low-fiber staples; when settled, ease back to soluble fiber like oats. For constipation, increase fluid and fiber gradually and walk when able; prunes or kiwi fruit can help. For early satiety, use smaller, more frequent meals with calorie-dense foods such as smoothies, nut butters, and olive oil.

Blood glucose and insulin resistance

Insulin is the hormone that moves glucose from your blood into your muscle and other tissues to be used for energy or stored. **Insulin resistance** occurs when those tissues stop responding properly. The body compensates by producing more insulin, but over time blood glucose rises. High blood sugar and high insulin together drive more inflammation, fatigue, and fat gain, particularly around the abdomen. In cancer, they are also associated with worse treatment tolerance and poorer survival.

Steroid medicines, which are often part of chemotherapy regimens, can temporarily raise blood glucose and worsen insulin resistance. Even outside of treatment, many people with cancer carry excess fat and low muscle mass — the exact combination that makes blood sugar control harder.

The good news is that both **diet** and **exercise** are powerful levers for improving insulin sensitivity. Small, repeatable habits add up quickly.

Practical dietary strategies

- **Build balanced plates.** Combine protein, healthy fats, and fiber-rich carbohydrates at each meal to slow digestion and prevent sharp glucose spikes.

- **Choose whole over refined.** Whole grains (oats, brown rice, quinoa, barley) release glucose more gradually than white bread, white rice, or sugary cereals.

- **Emphasize fiber.** Aim for 25–38 g/day. Soluble fiber (oats, beans, lentils, apples) is especially effective for stabilizing blood sugar.

- **Limit sugary drinks.** Sodas, fruit juice drinks, and energy drinks cause rapid spikes. Water, sparkling water, herbal teas, and milk/soy milk are better choices.

- **Spread carbohydrates through the day.** Divide carb foods across meals and snacks instead of loading them into one sitting.

- **Use protein and fat to steady responses.** Pair carbohydrate-rich foods with protein or healthy fat — for example, fruit with yoghurt or toast with nut butter.

- **Eat earlier in the day.** Glucose tolerance is better in the morning and midday than at night. Make breakfast and lunch your larger meals.

- **Include fermented foods.** Yoghurt, kefir, miso, sauerkraut, and kimchi support gut health, which influences glucose regulation.

Practical exercise strategies

- **Post-meal activity.** A 5–15 minute walk after meals lowers glucose by helping muscles absorb it directly. Pace can be gentle; consistency is key.

- **Resistance training.** Building muscle is one of the most effective long-term ways to improve insulin sensitivity. Even simple sit-to-stands, wall push-ups, or step-ups help.

- **Aerobic activity.** Walking, cycling, swimming, or dancing 20–30 minutes most days improves whole-body insulin sensitivity.

- **Break up sedentary time.** Stand, stretch, or walk briefly every 30–60 minutes to reduce glucose spikes.

- **Consistency matters.** Both resistance and aerobic training improve insulin sensitivity, but the effects fade after 2–3 days. Aim to move most days of the week.

Special considerations for people with cancer

- **During steroid treatment:** expect higher blood glucose, especially after meals. Focus on balanced plates, avoid sugary foods, and add a short walk after each meal if possible.

- **If appetite is poor:** choose small, nutrient-dense meals with protein and fiber, such as yoghurt with berries or lentil soup.

- **If underweight:** blood sugar control remains important, but priority is maintaining weight and muscle. Use calorie- and protein-dense foods, not sugary drinks.

- **If diabetic or pre-diabetic:** cancer treatment may alter medication needs. Work closely with both oncology and diabetes teams.

Hydration

Hydration is central to recovery, energy, and treatment tolerance. Treatments can change thirst, increase fluid losses, and alter kidney stress. Aim for steady intake through the day. Water, sparkling water, milk/soy milk, unsweetened tea or coffee, and broths all count. Flavoring water with citrus or herbs can help. Use electrolytes in hot weather, with diarrhea, or heavy sweating. Pale yellow urine is a practical guide to adequacy.

To emphasize, room or refrigerator temperature plain water is the best for body re-hydration. If you want to make a very effective and inexpensive "sports" drink then add some honey and a tiny amount of table salt!

Bone health

Hormone therapies such as androgen deprivation and aromatase inhibitors accelerate bone loss. Nutritional support includes adequate calcium (dairy, fortified plant milks, tofu set with calcium, leafy greens, nuts) and vitamin D guided by blood testing. Protein also supports bone by providing collagen building blocks. Combined with resistance and impact exercise, this is a key strategy for maintaining bone strength.

Managing side effects

Food can help with common side effects. For taste and smell changes, use plastic cutlery, lean on tart flavors, and consider cold meats to reduce aromas. For mouth sores, choose soft, cool foods and avoid stinging ingredients. Dry mouth improves with frequent sips and moist foods. Early satiety calls for smaller, calorie-dense meals. Constipation responds to fluids and gradual fiber; diarrhea requires rehydration and temporary low-fiber choices.

Cultural and access considerations

Mediterranean-style eating is well supported, but advice must fit cultural food traditions. Asian diets often emphasize rice, soy, and fish; South American diets legumes and maize; Middle Eastern diets pulses, flatbreads, and herbs—the principles translate. Cost and access matter. Frozen vegetables, canned beans, and tinned fish are nutritious, affordable, and safe. Local, seasonal foods are often best value. If possible, growing even a small pot of herbs or greens adds nutrition and pleasure.

Local and home-grown foods

Choosing foods grown close to home reduces storage time and nutrient loss. Local produce also carries microorganisms from your environment that may benefit the microbiome while reducing exposure to foreign microbes. If you can, grow some of your own food. Even a small window box of herbs, a tomato plant in a pot, or a trough of leafy greens improves diet quality and provides gentle physical activity and stress relief. Tomatoes, cruciferous vegetables, and leafy greens are particularly powerful additions and can be grown in small spaces.

Eating for mental health

Diet influences mood and cognition. Whole-food, plant-forward patterns with adequate omega-3s and fiber are consistently associated with lower depression and anxiety symptoms. Stable blood sugar and regular protein support energy and focus—critical during treatment and recovery.

Food safety during low counts

When blood counts drop, strict "neutropenic diets" have not shown added benefit. What matters is safe handling: wash hands and surfaces, separate raw and cooked foods, cook thoroughly, chill promptly, avoid raw sprouts and unpasteurized products, and steer clear of undercooked eggs or meats.

Working with medicines

Food–drug interactions matter. Grapefruit can alter how certain drugs are metabolized, raising blood levels. Warfarin interacts with vitamin K—aim for consistent intake rather than avoidance. Always tell your oncology team about supplements and herbal products; this is about safety, not permission.

Supplements: when "more" is not better

A basic multivitamin at recommended levels can be reasonable when appetite is poor. High-dose antioxidant supplements during chemotherapy are not recommended, as they may interfere with treatment. Vitamin D and B12 are important in selected cases. Omega-3 supplements have a role in selected cachexia settings; otherwise, a food-first approach is preferable.

Superfoods and practical choices

There is no single miracle food, but some foods consistently deliver more nutrition per bite and are easy to use day-to-day. Think of these as "high-leverage staples" rather than magic bullets, and rotate them through your week.

Berries are naturally sweet, high in fiber, and rich in antioxidants. Fresh or frozen, they are excellent in yoghurt, oats, smoothies, or eaten alone.

Fish provides protein and, in oily varieties like salmon, sardines, and mackerel, long-chain omega-3s. Fresh, frozen, or canned all work.

Leafy greens such as spinach, kale, and chard supply vitamins A and C, calcium, and phytochemicals. Add to soups, omelets, or sauté with olive oil

Cruciferous vegetables like broccoli, Brussels sprouts, and cabbage contain compounds linked with lower cancer risk. Steam, stir-fry, roast, or add frozen mixes to casseroles.

Legumes—beans, lentils, chickpeas, soybeans, peas—deliver protein, fiber, and folate. Use in soups, curries, salads, or spreads like hummus.

Whole grains provide fiber, B vitamins, and steady energy. Rotate oats, brown rice, quinoa, barley, and bulgur.

Nuts and seeds offer plant protein and healthy fats. A small handful daily is plenty; add to yoghurt, oats, or salads. Nut butters are also versatile.

Olive oil is a cornerstone of Mediterranean eating—use for sautéing, dressings, and drizzling.

Yoghurt with live cultures supplies protein and beneficial bacteria. Choose plain versions, add fruit, and use pasteurized products if counts are low.

Tomatoes, rich in vitamin C and lycopene, are even more beneficial when cooked with olive oil. Add to sauces, soups, and stews.

Buying close to home preserves nutrient content and supports your microbiome. Growing your own food—even just herbs in a pot—adds nutrition, activity, and relaxation. Tomatoes, cruciferous vegetables, and leafy greens are easy "superfoods" to grow.

Why people with cancer or in survivorship should avoid or minimize alcohol

Alcohol is now recognized as a Group 1 carcinogen by the World Health Organization — the same category as tobacco and asbestos. This means that there is strong evidence that alcohol can cause cancer. It does so by several mechanisms:

1. DNA damage: When alcohol is broken down in the body, it forms a toxic substance called *acetaldehyde*, which can damage DNA and make it harder for cells to repair themselves.
2. Hormone disruption: Alcohol increases levels of circulating estrogen and other hormones that can drive hormone-sensitive cancers such as breast, ovarian, and prostate cancer.
3. Oxidative stress and inflammation: Alcohol metabolism generates free radicals that can damage cells and tissues, promoting chronic inflammation — a key process in cancer growth and progression.
4. Impaired immune function: Even moderate drinking can suppress immune defenses, making it harder for the body to detect and destroy cancer cells.
5. Interference with treatment and recovery: Alcohol can worsen side effects of chemotherapy, immunotherapy, or radiation (for example, fatigue, nausea, neuropathy, or liver stress) and can interfere with medications used during or after treatment.

During cancer treatment

Alcohol places extra strain on the liver, which is already working hard to process chemotherapy and other drugs. It can worsen mouth sores, dehydration, nausea, and fatigue, and can interfere with sleep and healing. Even small amounts may affect balance, mood, and judgement, especially when combined with medications.

In survivorship

Alcohol use is linked to higher risk of cancer recurrence and new primary cancers, particularly breast, mouth, throat, liver, and bowel cancers. It also contributes to other chronic conditions common after cancer treatment, such as cardiovascular disease, diabetes, and osteoporosis. Because alcohol provides "empty calories", it can lead to unwanted weight gain and central obesity, which are also associated with poorer cancer outcomes.

What's the safest amount?

The latest international guidelines (e.g., WHO, Cancer Council Australia, and the American Cancer Society) are very clear:

The safest level of alcohol for people with cancer is zero. If you choose to drink, less is better — ideally no more than 1 standard drink on occasional days, and none most of the time.

The bottom line

Avoiding or greatly minimizing alcohol supports your body's recovery, strengthens your immune system, helps maintain a healthy weight, improves sleep and energy, and reduces the risk of recurrence or new cancers. Combined with good nutrition and regular exercise, it's one of the simplest and most powerful lifestyle choices for long-term survivorship.

Gentle guardrails

- Aim for 1.2–1.6 g/kg/day of protein spread across three or four meals.
- Let plants fill most of your plate most of the time.
- Favor olive oil, nuts, seeds, avocado, and fish; limit processed fats.
- Keep red meat modest and processed meats minimal.
- Keep alcohol low or avoid it especially during treatments and recovery. Try to consume modestly during survivorship.
- Practice safe food handling during low blood cell counts.
- Use mindful eating to reduce distracted over- or under-eating. Don't eat in front of television or your phone.

Nutrition priorities at a glance

Focus area	During treatment	After treatment / survivorship
Primary goal	Maintain weight and strength; prevent malnutrition	Optimize body composition (reduce excess fat, protect/gain muscle)
Protein	≥1.2–1.6 g/kg/day; spread across meals; use soft, easy options if appetite is low	1.2–1.6 g/kg/day; up to 2.0 g/kg if rebuilding muscle
Energy	Eat enough to prevent unplanned weight loss; small, frequent meals if appetite is low	If safe, modest deficit (0.25–0.5 kg/week) for fat loss while protecting muscle
Carbohydrate & fiber	Whole grains, fruits, vegetables as tolerated; adjust fiber for bowel symptoms	25–38 g/day fiber from plants and whole grains; stabilize blood sugar
Fats	Olive oil, nuts, seeds, avocado, oily fish; reduce ultra-processed fats	Same pattern long-term
Hydration	Steady fluids; broths, milk/soy milk, herbal teas; electrolytes if vomiting/diarrhea or heat	Maintain hydration; water as main fluid; limit sugary drinks and alcohol
Microbiome support	Prebiotics (oats, legumes, whole grains); food-based probiotics (yoghurt, kefir, miso; pasteurized if counts low)	Continue varied prebiotic fiber and fermented foods; greater diversity supports resilience

Focus area	During treatment	After treatment / survivorship
Food safety	Strict safe handling; avoid raw sprouts, unpasteurized products, undercooked meat/eggs	Standard safe handling; no blanket restrictions
Inflammation	Plant-forward eating; minimize processed meats and refined foods	Continue Mediterranean-style pattern
Side effects	Soft, cool foods for mucositis; bland choices for nausea; adjust fiber for bowel changes	Restore variety and fiber gradually
Weight management	Weight loss generally not advised; prioritize maintaining muscle	Gentle fat loss if appropriate; always pair with protein and resistance training
Supplements	Only if indicated (Vit D, B12, omega-3 in cachexia); avoid high-dose antioxidants during chemo	Supplements for documented deficiencies; food-first approach

Nutrition does not need to be complicated to be effective.

Build a reliable pattern that supports exercise medicine: enough protein and energy, mostly plants, simple meals you enjoy, and flexible strategies for hard days. From that base, we can fine-tune for treatment, recovery, and long-term health.

CHAPTER 24

Precision Nutrition: The Next Frontier in Nutritional Medicine

Despite what I just said at the end of the previous chapter…

The next frontier in nutritional medicine is precision nutrition — tailoring what, when, and how we eat to match the biology of each individual and their cancer. Just as oncologists now match drugs to tumor subtypes and genetic mutations, nutrition science is learning to match food and nutrient strategies to a person's genes, metabolism, microbiome, and treatment context. For people with cancer and in survivorship, this represents a shift from one-size-fits-all advice toward a truly personalized approach.

Precision nutrition builds upon the healthy eating foundations already described in this chapter. It does not replace Mediterranean-style or plant-forward patterns, but rather refines them by asking a more targeted question: *What version of this pattern works best for you, at this moment, given your unique biology and treatment?*

What precision nutrition means in cancer care

Cancer is not a single disease. Each tumor type — and even each patient's version of that tumor — has its own metabolic fingerprint. Some cancers thrive on glucose, others depend heavily on certain amino acids or fats. Treatments such as chemotherapy, immunotherapy, or hormone therapy also alter metabolism in distinct ways. Precision nutrition aims to understand these variables and design dietary strategies that complement medical treatment, reduce side effects, and improve resilience.

At its core, precision nutrition involves three layers of information:

- **Host biology** — your genes, metabolism, hormones, and body composition.

- **Tumor biology** — the specific molecular and metabolic traits of your cancer.
- **Lifestyle and environment** — including your microbiome, activity levels, and daily rhythms of eating and sleeping.

When these layers are integrated, diet can be used not only to support overall health but to enhance treatment response and long-term recovery.

Moving from population averages to personal data

For decades, dietary guidelines were built on population averages — the best advice for most people most of the time. But patients differ greatly in how they process food. Two people can eat identical meals and show completely different blood sugar and insulin responses. These differences stem from genetics, gut bacteria, muscle mass, sleep patterns, and even the time of day the meal is eaten. Precision nutrition uses these data to predict and personalize responses, allowing dietary prescriptions to be as individual as a fingerprint.

In clinical research, machine-learning models that combine genetic, metabolic, and microbiome information can now predict which foods stabilize glucose for each person. Similar approaches are emerging in oncology. For example, ongoing trials are testing whether diets tailored to a patient's metabolic and microbiome profile can improve weight control and blood sugar during endocrine therapy for breast cancer. Early findings suggest that such personalization helps maintain treatment response while improving energy and body composition.

Genes, metabolism, and nutrient pathways

Certain genetic variations can change how nutrients are metabolized. For example, people with differences in folate-handling or antioxidant genes may need higher intakes of leafy greens or cruciferous vegetables to maintain optimal DNA repair and detoxification. Others with genetic tendencies toward insulin resistance often respond better to lower-glycemic diets and higher physical activity.

Nutrigenomics — how nutrients influence gene expression — is equally important. Bioactive compounds in foods such as soy (genistein), turmeric (curcumin), and broccoli (sulforaphane) can turn on tumor-suppressor genes and dampen inflammation. These effects are subtle but meaningful, especially when combined with exercise, which triggers many of the same protective pathways.

Tumor metabolism and targeted dietary strategies

Emerging research shows that tumors vary in their nutrient preferences. Some fast-growing cancers, such as triple-negative and HER2-positive breast cancers, rely heavily on glucose. For these, short cycles of fasting or fasting-mimicking diets may lower circulating glucose and insulin, making cancer cells more vulnerable to treatment while protecting normal cells. Other tumors depend on specific amino acids, such as methionine or serine; restricting these nutrients under medical supervision is being tested as a way to slow tumor growth and enhance chemotherapy.

In hormone-sensitive cancers, such as many breast and prostate cancers, the goal is often to reduce fat-driven estrogen and androgen production. Here, modest calorie control, high fiber intake, and regular physical activity — particularly resistance training — help reduce body fat and stabilize hormones. For every subtype, maintaining muscle mass remains critical; muscle is not only a metabolic organ but also a buffer against inflammation and fatigue.

The microbiome connection

The gut microbiome acts as a control center linking diet, immunity, and treatment response. A diverse gut ecosystem supports better tolerance to chemotherapy and stronger responses to immunotherapy. Diets rich in fiber, colorful plants, and fermented foods foster this diversity. Precision nutrition seeks to map each person's microbiome and guide dietary changes that restore balance — for example, adjusting fiber type or fermented food intake based on microbial composition. Over time, these tailored approaches will enhance both treatment effectiveness and psychological wellbeing.

Precision nutrition and exercise medicine

Precision nutrition and exercise medicine are two halves of the same system. Both target metabolism, inflammation, and immune health. Exercise increases insulin sensitivity and muscle glucose uptake; nutrition provides the substrates for repair and recovery. When combined, they create an environment less favorable to cancer progression and more supportive of energy, mood, and functional independence.

For instance, timing carbohydrate intake around exercise sessions can stabilize blood sugar and reduce fatigue. Adequate protein after training supports muscle synthesis, while plant-based polyphenols and omega-3 fats reduce post-exercise inflammation. These adjustments are simple examples of precision nutrition in everyday practice — matching fuel to function.

From laboratory to daily life

While precision nutrition draws on complex science — genomics, metabolomics, and microbiome analysis — its application can be practical. Continuous glucose monitors, wearable sensors, and smartphone apps now allow patients to see how food and activity interact in real time. Small experiments — trying different meal timings, adjusting carbohydrate sources, or testing overnight fasting — can help individuals learn what supports their energy, mood, and sleep best during recovery.

As the evidence base grows, oncologists and dietitians will increasingly use biomarkers — such as insulin, inflammatory markers, and microbial metabolites — to fine-tune dietary advice alongside treatment. The ultimate aim is not dietary perfection but a personalized pattern that fits your biology and your life.

Looking ahead

Precision nutrition represents the next evolution in cancer survivorship care. It combines the wisdom of whole-food, plant-based eating with cutting-edge insights from genetics, metabolism, and digital health. It asks not just *what* to eat, but *who* is eating it, *when*, and *why*. For patients, it means a shift from generic rules to guided experimentation — a partnership between science, clinician, and individual experience.

In time, precision nutrition will enable dietary strategies to be prescribed as confidently as medicines: evidence-based, monitored, and adapted as your needs change through treatment and beyond. For now, the message is both simple and empowering — learn your body, track your responses, and work with your clinicians to align your food, exercise, and treatment plan. Nutrition is not an accessory to cancer care; it is part of the precision medicine revolution that is reshaping it.

A final word I tell every patient

Food is not a cure. But used wisely, it is powerful support. It helps you keep muscle quantity and quality, limit fat mass, steady energy balance, and makes exercise medicine work better. Start where you are. Choose one or two changes from this chapter and live with them for a week. Then choose one or two more. If you hit a snag—or if the scale moves faster than feels safe—circle back with your team and your oncology dietitian. This is a long game, and you're not playing it alone.

CHAPTER 25

Exercise and the Immune System

Your immune system is your body's security and repair network. Every day, billions of cells patrol your bloodstream, lymphatic system, and tissues—searching for infection, clearing damaged cells, and destroying abnormal ones before they can form tumors. Cancer can develop when this system falters or when rogue cells find ways to hide from immune detection. Treatments such as chemotherapy and radiation can weaken immunity, leaving people more vulnerable to infection and fatigue. The exciting discovery from modern research is that exercise can strengthen and re-train this system. When you move your body, you activate natural defense mechanisms that make it harder for cancer to thrive. Exercise is not an external drug—it's a way of producing internal medicine that works in harmony with your biology.

How Exercise Interacts with the Immune System

The immune system has two major arms: innate immunity, which provides rapid first-line defense, and adaptive immunity, which learns and remembers. Exercise influences both. Each session mobilizes billions of immune cells, improves blood and lymph flow, reduces inflammation, and recalibrates stress hormones that otherwise suppress immunity. The result is an environment where your immune system becomes more vigilant, balanced, and efficient.

In healthy people, these effects help prevent infection and chronic disease. In people living with or beyond cancer, they go even further—helping the immune system recognize and destroy cancer cells, improving tolerance to treatment, and speeding recovery. Unlike drugs that target one pathway, exercise works across the entire network: muscle, bone marrow, blood, lymph nodes, gut, and even the brain communicate to fine-tune defense.

Acute Immune Activation – What Happens During a Single Exercise Session

When you start moving, your body responds immediately. Heart rate and breathing rise, and so does blood flow through the muscles and organs. This rapid circulation is sensed by immune cells resting along vessel walls. Adrenaline and noradrenaline surge, acting as a "wake-up call." These hormones tell natural killer (NK) cells, cytotoxic T-cells, and monocytes to enter the bloodstream. Within minutes, immune cell numbers can increase tenfold.

These mobilized cells are not passive passengers—they are primed for action. NK cells are the body's fast-response assassins. They can detect and destroy abnormal cells without needing prior exposure. During and shortly after exercise, NK cells travel through the body, scanning tissues for trouble. Research shows that in this window—roughly the first hour after moderate-to-vigorous exercise—tumor cells in laboratory models are more likely to be attacked and destroyed. The same process likely occurs at a smaller scale in humans: regular bouts of exercise repeatedly flush active immune cells through the body's tissues, including tumors, improving surveillance and clearance.

This acute response fades after a few hours as the stress hormones normalize, but that's not a sign of suppression—it's part of the cycle. Immune cells migrate into tissues, perform their duties, and return to resting pools better trained for the next challenge. Each session acts like a rehearsal for the immune system, building efficiency without causing exhaustion.

Chronic Adaptations – How Regular Exercise Strengthens Immunity

When these short-term immune activations are repeated consistently, long-term remodeling occurs. The immune system becomes more balanced and less prone to chronic inflammation—the smoldering background fire that can promote cancer growth and fatigue.

Chronic low-grade inflammation is common in cancer and aging. It's driven by excess fat tissue, stress hormones, and physical inactivity.

Exercise turns down this inflammatory noise through several mechanisms:

1. Reduction of visceral fat, which produces harmful inflammatory cytokines.

2. Release of myokines—hormone-like molecules from contracting muscles—that act as anti-inflammatory messengers.

3. Improved autonomic balance, lowering cortisol and sympathetic stress responses that otherwise suppress immune function.

4. Enhanced antioxidant capacity, protecting immune cells from oxidative damage caused by treatments or metabolic stress.

Over weeks and months, regular exercise leads to a healthier balance between pro-inflammatory and anti-inflammatory signals. The result is a system that is alert but not overactive—able to fight threats without causing collateral damage.

These changes are visible in measurable ways. People who exercise regularly show greater numbers of naïve T-cells (the "rookies" ready to learn new targets) and fewer exhausted or senescent T-cells that have lost their effectiveness. Antibody responses to vaccines improve. Wound healing is faster. In cancer survivors, this translates to better tolerance of therapy, fewer infections, and potentially improved tumor control.

Exercise and the Microbiome – Training the Inner Ecosystem

Over the past decade, research has revealed a hidden partner in exercise medicine: the trillions of microbes that live along our digestive tract. This microscopic community—known as the gut microbiome—acts like a vast chemical factory and immune-training ground. It produces vitamins, hormones, and short-chain fatty acids that calm inflammation, regulate metabolism, and communicate directly with immune cells.

When the microbiome is diverse and balanced, it supports health at every level. When it becomes imbalanced or depleted—a state called dysbiosis—immune regulation falters, inflammation rises, and the effectiveness of many cancer treatments declines. Chemotherapy, radiation, antibiotics, and stress can all disrupt this fragile ecosystem. Exercise helps restore it.

1. How Exercise Shapes the Microbiome

Every bout of moderate to vigorous physical activity increases blood flow to the intestines and stimulates rhythmic contractions that mix and move intestinal contents. This gentle mechanical motion improves oxygen delivery and nutrient exchange for the microbes that live there. Regular exercise also raises the abundance of beneficial bacterial species such as *Faecalibacterium prausnitzii* and *Akkermansia muciniphila*—organisms linked with anti-inflammatory metabolites and enhanced immune tolerance.

At the same time, exercise reduces the overgrowth of species that thrive on sedentary behavior, high-fat, or highly processed diets. The overall effect is greater microbial diversity—a broader range of "voices" in the immune conversation. In both animal and human studies, people who exercise regularly show higher levels of short-chain fatty acids such as butyrate, acetate, and propionate. These compounds nourish colon cells, seal the gut barrier, and send calming signals throughout the immune system.

2. The Gut–Immune–Brain Axis

The microbiome communicates constantly with the brain and immune system through neural, hormonal, and chemical channels. When the gut environment is healthy, it produces molecules that reduce systemic inflammation and influence mood and cognition. This explains why many patients describe improved mental clarity and emotional stability after establishing an exercise routine—the benefit travels not only through the muscles and heart but also through the gut–brain axis.

Exercise reinforces this loop by lowering stress hormones that would otherwise disrupt intestinal balance. Cortisol and adrenaline in excess thin the gut lining and change microbial populations; regular exercise reverses that pattern. The result is a calmer immune system and a steadier emotional state.

3. Implications for Cancer Therapy

A balanced microbiome enhances the effectiveness of chemotherapy, radiation, and especially immunotherapy. Studies show that patients with richer microbial diversity respond better to immune checkpoint inhibitors and experience fewer severe side effects. Exercise, by improving gut health and circulation, indirectly primes the immune system for these therapies.

I often explain it this way: when you exercise, you are not only strengthening your muscles—you are training an entire internal ecosystem to work on your behalf. The gut becomes a communication hub, sending biochemical messages that say “heal,” “repair,” and “stay balanced.”

4. Practical Ways to Support the Gut Through Exercise

- **Combine exercise with a plant-forward diet.** Fiber from fruits, vegetables, legumes, and whole grains feeds the microbes that produce beneficial short-chain fatty acids.
- **Stay hydrated.** Adequate fluid keeps the digestive tract moving and supports microbial metabolism.
- **Manage stress and sleep.** Overtraining or chronic stress can undo the gains; balance effort with recovery.
- **Use antibiotics only when essential.** If treatment requires them, restore microbial diversity afterward through food variety, probiotics, and consistent physical activity.

5. The Take-Home Message

Your gut microbiome is a living organ in its own right—one that responds dynamically to exercise. Every step, every breath, and every contraction sends a positive signal to this internal community. By moving your body, you are cultivating a microbiome that, in turn, strengthens your immunity, improves your mood, and enhances your response to cancer treatment.

The muscle and the microbe are partners in the same therapy—each supporting the other to build a stronger, more resilient host.

Exercise and Cancer Therapies – Synergy in Action

The relationship between exercise and medical treatment is not competition—it's collaboration. Exercise can enhance the effectiveness of chemotherapy, radiation, and immunotherapy by changing the internal environment in which these treatments work.

Chemotherapy: Many drugs rely on adequate blood flow and oxygen to reach tumor sites. Exercise temporarily increases tumor perfusion and oxygenation, making drug delivery more uniform. At the same time, improved immune function helps clear damaged cells and supports bone marrow recovery between cycles.

Radiation Therapy: Radiation kills cells by generating reactive oxygen species. Tumors with better oxygen supply facilitate radiation effectiveness. Exercise before radiation sessions can improve oxygen delivery to the tumor microenvironment, potentially enhancing treatment precision while protecting healthy tissue through improved circulation and antioxidant defense.

Immunotherapy: Drugs such as immune checkpoint inhibitors work by reactivating exhausted T-cells. Exercise amplifies this effect by increasing the number and activity of these cells. It also improves the diversity of the gut microbiome—a factor now known to influence immunotherapy response. Regular physical activity may therefore help immunotherapy work better and with fewer side effects.

Targeted and Hormonal Therapies: These treatments often alter metabolism and body composition, leading to insulin resistance and inflammation that blunt immune efficiency. Exercise directly counteracts these effects, maintaining metabolic and immune resilience.

The combined result is that exercise does not merely make patients "fitter"—it makes the body a more favorable partner for medical therapy. Think of it as recalibrating your internal environment to help modern oncology work at its best.

Practical Application – How to Train for Immune Health

Immune benefits arise from both aerobic and resistance exercise. The key is regularity and moderation. Extreme training or prolonged exhaustive exercise can temporarily suppress immunity, but the levels recommended in cancer care are well below that threshold.

Frequency: Aim for activity on most days—ideally five or more per week. Even brief sessions count; the immune system responds to exercise, not just duration.

Intensity: Moderate to moderately hard effort is ideal. On the 0–10 perceived exertion scale, that means about 4–6. You should breathe faster but still be able to speak in short sentences. For those who enjoy numbers, this corresponds to roughly 60–70% of heart-rate reserve.

Duration: Twenty to forty minutes of continuous aerobic exercise, or several shorter bouts totaling 30–60 minutes per day, is sufficient. For resistance training, two to three sessions per week covering major muscle groups provides strong immune and metabolic benefits.

Modes: Walking, cycling, swimming, stepping, or low-impact circuit training all work well. Include resistance exercises such as squats, deadlifts, presses, or rows to engage large muscle groups—the body's primary "myokine factories."

Consistency: Regular moderate sessions outperform infrequent vigorous bursts. The immune system thrives on rhythm. A short daily walk or strength session is better than a single long workout followed by several sedentary days.

Timing Around Treatments: If possible, schedule light to moderate exercise a few hours before chemotherapy or radiation. Before treatment, improved circulation and oxygenation can enhance delivery; after treatment, fatigue may limit performance. On recovery days, gentle exercise like stretching or slow walking maintains blood and lymph flow.

Special Considerations

Infection Risk and Low Counts: During chemotherapy, blood counts can drop, reducing infection resistance. Light indoor exercise—stretching, breathing work, gentle cycling, or short walks—remains safe and beneficial, provided temperature, hydration, and hygiene are managed. Avoid crowded gyms and public pools when neutrophil counts are very low or when there is fever. Once counts recover, gradually return to full training.

Post-Surgery or Catheter Care: Exercise supports lymph flow and recovery but avoid heavy lifting or upper-body strain near surgical sites or lines until cleared. Gentle lower-body and breathing exercises are encouraged as early as possible to prevent deconditioning.

Fever, Severe Fatigue, or Chest Pain: These are red flags to pause exercise and contact your care team. Exercise enhances immunity when the body is stable, not when fighting acute infection.

Autoimmune Conditions: If you have coexisting autoimmune disease, exercise remains beneficial but should be titrated carefully. Gentle, consistent activity lowers inflammatory markers and improves joint and muscle health without triggering flares.

Sleep, Nutrition, and Stress: Exercise is most effective when paired with restorative sleep, adequate protein, and balanced stress management. Chronic sleep deprivation or poor diet blunts immune adaptation.

Key Takeaways

- Every session of moderate exercise mobilizes billions of immune cells, improving cancer surveillance.
- Regular training reduces chronic inflammation and supports bone marrow and lymph function.
- Exercise enhances the effectiveness of chemotherapy, radiation, and immunotherapy by improving oxygenation and immune readiness.
- Moderate intensity—about a 4–6 on the 0–10 exertion scale—is optimal for immune benefits.

- Combine aerobic and resistance training for the strongest effect.
- Moderate exercise is safe during treatment unless fever, severe fatigue, or very low blood counts occur.
- Light to moderate exercise (autoregulated), hydration, sleep, and balanced nutrition sustain immune recovery between treatments.
- Consistent exercise transforms your immune system into an active partner in cancer defense.

Exercise is not merely rehabilitation—it is immune re-education. Every time you move, you remind your body how to defend itself.

CHAPTER 26
Exercise for Mental Health, Cognitive Function and Sexual Health

Cancer affects the mind as profoundly as it affects the body. Anxiety, low mood, disrupted sleep, and cognitive fog are among the most common and distressing effects of both the disease and its treatments. Many people describe difficulty concentrating, slower thinking, forgetfulness, or a sense of mental heaviness. These symptoms can arise during treatment and persist for months or years.

Exercise is one of the most effective strategies to protect and restore mental health, cognitive clarity, and sexual wellbeing during and after cancer treatment. It influences brain chemistry, improves blood flow to the brain, reduces inflammation, stabilizes stress hormones, and supports the body's endocrine and neural systems. Exercise also restores a sense of capability and confidence that illness can erode.

In this chapter I explain how exercise improves mood and cognitive function, and how it contributes to restoring sexual health, intimacy, and bodily confidence in both women and men.

How Exercise Changes the Brain

Healthy brain function depends on balanced blood flow, oxygen supply, neural signaling, immune regulation, and chemical stability. Cancer treatments can disrupt these processes. Chemotherapy alters neurotransmitter pathways, radiation affects small blood vessels, endocrine therapy changes hormonal communication, disease and treatment increase oxidative stress, and chronic stress amplifies inflammation.

Exercise counteracts these disruptions. Contracting muscle releases chemical signals called myokines and hormones that travel to the brain and support cellular repair. Exercise increases brain-derived neurotrophic factor, an important molecule for the growth of new neurons and the strengthening of neural connections. This is particularly important in the hippocampus, the brain region responsible for memory, learning, and emotional regulation.

Aerobic exercise increases blood flow to the brain and enhances energy metabolism. Regular training improves the resilience of the microvasculature, helping to protect against treatment-related cognitive decline. Through these pathways, exercise restores and strengthens brain function at every level.

Mood, Stress, and Emotional Resilience

Cancer places significant psychological strain on the body. The uncertainty of diagnosis, treatment demands, and fear of recurrence activate the stress response system and elevate cortisol and adrenaline. When these hormones remain high for long periods, sleep worsens, anxiety increases, and immune function declines.

Exercise stabilizes this system. Even one session of moderate-intensity exercise increases endorphins, dopamine, serotonin, and other natural chemicals that lift mood and reduce pain. With regular training, the stress system becomes more balanced, cortisol surges are smaller, and the body returns to baseline more quickly.

Exercise also restores a sense of control. Completing an exercise session, even a brief one, provides clear evidence that you can influence your physical and emotional state. This shift from passive coping to active participation is one of the strongest psychological benefits of exercise medicine.

Exercise as Therapy for Depression and Anxiety

Exercise is an effective treatment for depression, but the type and intensity matter. Research shows that high-intensity progressive resistance training is the most powerful exercise-based therapy for clinical depression. The demanding nature of heavy lifting produces strong biological signals that regulate mood, including changes in neurotransmitters, hormonal pathways, and inflammatory processes. Strength gains themselves are associated with reductions in depressive symptoms. This form of training is safe with appropriate supervision and is particularly valuable for older adults, who may have limited tolerance for antidepressant medication.

Aerobic exercise is especially effective for anxiety. Rhythmic exercise, controlled breathing, and increased parasympathetic activity reduce physical tension and calm the mind. Even short sessions, such as a brief walk or cycle, can interrupt acute anxiety.

Together, resistance training and aerobic exercise form a comprehensive therapeutic approach. Resistance training provides the strongest antidepressant effect, while aerobic activity reduces anxiety, improves emotional regulation, and enhances sleep. Both modalities improve energy, confidence, and overall psychological resilience.

Exercise and Cognitive Function

Cognitive difficulties during or after treatment arise from inflammation, hormonal disruption, fatigue, stress, and changes in blood flow. Exercise improves each of these factors. Increased blood flow enhances delivery of oxygen and nutrients to the brain. Lower inflammation protects neural cells. Higher neurotrophic signaling improves learning, attention, and memory. Aerobic exercise tends to produce the most pronounced improvements in overall cognitive function, while resistance training assists through better sleep and hormonal stability.

Many people notice clearer thinking and improved concentration within weeks of starting regular exercise.

The Muscle–Brain Connection in Cognitive Impairment

Newer research shows that some of the cognitive problems linked with chemotherapy begin outside the brain, in skeletal muscle. Chemotherapy can damage the mitochondria inside muscle cells. When mitochondria are impaired, muscle fibers release higher levels of inflammatory molecules and oxidative by-products into the bloodstream. These circulating signals reach the brain and trigger a second wave of inflammation and oxidative stress, particularly in regions responsible for memory and executive function.

This creates a feedback loop where muscle dysfunction amplifies brain dysfunction. Even if chemotherapy drugs do not enter the brain directly, the stress signals originating from damaged muscle can impair neurogenesis, disrupt mitochondrial function in neurons, and contribute to slower thinking, forgetfulness, and reduced mental clarity.

Exercise interrupts this loop. It restores mitochondrial health in muscle, reduces the inflammatory and oxidative signals entering the bloodstream, and increases myokines such as brain-derived neurotrophic factor and irisin, which support neuronal repair. These changes help protect the brain from treatment-related cognitive effects and improve its ability to recover.

Social and Behavioral Benefits

Exercise provides routine, structure, and connection. Group classes, walking programs, or supervised exercise sessions offer support and accountability. These elements reduce isolation and increase motivation during treatment and recovery. Exercise also restores daily rhythm, supporting appetite, sleep, and energy balance. For many people, this becomes an anchor of stability during uncertain times.

Sexual Health and Intimacy After Cancer

Sexual health is an important contributor to quality of life, yet it is often overlooked in cancer care. Treatments can change libido, arousal, lubrication, erectile function, continence, body image, and comfort with intimacy. These effects influence identity, confidence, and emotional connection.

Exercise plays a meaningful role in restoring sexual health in both women and men. It supports vascular function, hormonal stability, neuromuscular control, body composition, psychological wellbeing, and pelvic-floor strength. It also helps people reconnect with their bodies and regain confidence in physical closeness.

Sexual Health in Women

Women experience changes in sexual function through multiple pathways. Chemotherapy, endocrine therapy, pelvic radiation, surgery, and therapy-induced menopause can affect libido, arousal, lubrication, vaginal comfort, pelvic-floor control, and body image. Vaginal dryness and discomfort are common. Sensitivity may change after breast or pelvic surgery. Fatigue, anxiety, and altered body perception can further reduce sexual desire and enjoyment.

A large clinical trial in women with metastatic breast cancer showed that supervised exercise improved sexual functioning and enjoyment and reduced vaginal symptoms compared with usual care. Women who exercised experienced improved lubrication, reduced discomfort, and greater ease of arousal.

Exercise supports women's sexual health through several mechanisms:

- improved genital blood flow and enhanced tissue oxygenation
- increased lubrication and reduced vaginal dryness
- reduced pain and discomfort during sexual activity
- improved pelvic-floor strength, neuromuscular control, and continence
- reduced systemic inflammation and improved vaginal tissue health
- improved body composition, posture, and physical capability
- increased energy and less treatment-related fatigue
- improved mood, reduced anxiety, and better emotional regulation
- enhanced body image, confidence, and comfort with physical closeness

These mechanisms help restore arousal, pleasure, and comfort, contributing to a fuller sense of sexual and relational confidence.

Sexual Health in Men

Men undergoing prostate cancer treatment, particularly androgen suppression, often face substantial sexual health challenges. Libido decreases, erectile function declines, muscle mass falls, fat increases, and continence may be affected. These changes influence identity and confidence as much as physical function.

Exercise provides a pathway to recovery. Resistance and aerobic training improve erectile function, restore lean mass, reduce fat, and enhance circulation. Improved pelvic-floor strength supports continence and confidence during intimacy. Exercise also improves mood, reduces anxiety, and restores a sense of physical competence.

Clinical trials show that structured exercise improves erectile function, intercourse satisfaction, and overall sexual activity, even in men receiving hormone suppression. Many men describe feeling more physically capable and more connected to their bodies as strength and vitality return.

Exercise Supports Men's Sexual Health Through:

- improved erectile function via enhanced vascular and endothelial health
- increased nitric oxide availability and improved genital blood flow
- reversal of treatment-related body changes through increased lean mass and reduced fat mass
- improved pelvic-floor and core strength, supporting urinary control and sexual confidence
- increased testosterone signaling and androgen receptor sensitivity (even during hormone therapy)
- reduced inflammation and better metabolic health
- improved vitality, energy, and reduced fatigue
- reduced anxiety and depressive symptoms
- improved masculine self-esteem, body image, and sense of physical capability

These mechanisms help men regain sexual function, desire, performance confidence, and intimate connection.

Practical Strategies

- **Aerobic exercise:** improves arousal, anxiety regulation, mood stability, and vascular function.
- **Resistance training:** provides the strongest antidepressant effect, builds lean mass, improves body image and libido, and enhances pelvic stability.
- **Pelvic-floor and core strengthening:** improves continence and physical control, supporting comfort during intimacy.
- **Flexibility and mobility work:** improves ease of movement and reduces discomfort during sexual activity.
- **Consistency:** regular exercise produces cumulative improvements in mood, cognition, and sexual wellbeing.
- **Supportive environment:** exercising with others or in a welcoming clinic reduces fear and increases confidence.

Key Takeaways

- Exercise improves mood, reduces anxiety, and restores clarity of thought.
- High-intensity resistance training is a powerful therapy for clinical depression.
- Aerobic exercise is especially effective for anxiety and emotional regulation.
- Exercise enhances sexual health in both women and men by improving vascular, hormonal, neural, and psychological pathways.

Consistency is essential. Even small sessions contribute to recovery. Exercise supports identity, confidence, and connection.

Exercise is both physical and psychological medicine. It strengthens the body, steadies the mind, and restores confidence and intimacy during and after cancer treatment.

CHAPTER 27

Cardio-Oncology: Protecting the Heart and Circulatory System

Cancer treatment places unique demands on the cardiovascular system. The heart, which beats more than 100,000 times each day, supplies oxygen and nutrients to every organ. During cancer therapy, this finely tuned engine can be challenged by chemotherapy, targeted therapies, radiation, hormonal manipulation, metabolic disruption, and the psychological burden of the diagnosis. Cardio-oncology is the field that examines how cancer and its treatments affect the heart and circulation, and how to prevent or manage these effects.

The encouraging reality is that exercise offers powerful protection. It strengthens the heart, improves vascular function, enhances cardiorespiratory fitness, counteracts treatment-related metabolic changes, and supports long-term cardiovascular resilience. In this chapter I explain how cancer therapies influence the cardiovascular system, how exercise provides systemic protection, and how to train safely and effectively during and after treatment.

How Cancer and Its Treatments Affect the Heart

Cancer itself, along with the physical and emotional stress of diagnosis and therapy, influences cardiovascular health. Inflammation, oxidative stress, changes in hormone levels, fatigue, and metabolic disruptions all contribute. Several treatments carry specific cardiovascular effects.

Anthracycline Chemotherapy

Drugs such as doxorubicin and epirubicin can damage mitochondria and contractile fibers in heart muscle cells. At high cumulative doses these changes may reduce pumping efficiency or, in rare cases, lead to heart failure.

HER2-Targeted Therapies

Agents such as trastuzumab and pertuzumab may cause temporary reductions in heart function. These effects are usually reversible with early detection and management.

Radiation Therapy

Radiation to the chest or left breast can expose parts of the heart and coronary arteries to small scatter doses. Over years this can contribute to stiffness, inflammation, or accelerated plaque formation.

Hormone and Targeted Therapies

Androgen deprivation therapy in men and aromatase inhibitors in women can increase fat mass, reduce muscle mass, alter cholesterol, and impair glucose control. Some targeted agents raise blood pressure or cause fluid retention. These changes increase cardiovascular strain.

Cardiovascular Injury Extends Beyond the Heart

Treatment-related cardiotoxicity affects more than the heart muscle. Cancer therapies can injure the entire cardiorespiratory and muscular system, including the vascular endothelium, skeletal muscle mitochondria, pulmonary tissue, the autonomic nervous system, and metabolic organs. These systems work together to support cardiac reserve, and injury to any one of them reduces overall cardiovascular resilience.

For example, chemotherapy can impair skeletal muscle mitochondria, lowering energy production and increasing oxidative stress. Radiation can stiffen the chest wall and lungs, altering breathing mechanics. Hormone therapy worsens metabolic health, increasing cardiovascular load. Autonomic dysregulation can reduce heart-rate control and slow recovery after exertion.

Because exercise influences each of these systems, it is uniquely positioned to repair and strengthen the full network involved in cardiovascular function.

Why Cardiorespiratory Fitness Predicts Long-Term Outcomes

Resting cardiac imaging often appears normal even when physiological reserve is reduced. The limitation is not always in the heart's pumping ability at rest, but in its capacity to increase output during exertion. This reserve is reflected in peak oxygen uptake (VO_2peak), which integrates heart function, lung capacity, blood flow, oxygen-carrying capacity, skeletal muscle mitochondrial function, and autonomic control.

VO_2peak is one of the strongest predictors of long-term survival in cancer survivors. Even small increases achieved through structured training reduce cardiovascular events and mortality. Exercise is the most effective way to raise VO_2peak and restore cardiac reserve.

How Exercise Protects the Heart and Circulatory System

Exercise strengthens the heart and optimizes the function of the vessels that supply it. These adaptations improve treatment tolerance and long-term health.

Improved Pumping Capacity

Aerobic exercise increases stroke volume and lowers resting heart rate, making the heart more efficient and resilient.

Improved Coronary Circulation

Exercise increases blood flow through the coronary arteries and stimulates the growth of new micro vessels, improving oxygen delivery even in areas with partial narrowing.

Improved Vascular Function

Exercise enhances endothelial responsiveness and arterial elasticity. This lowers blood pressure and reduces clot risk.

Cellular Protection

Exercise increases antioxidant capacity and mitochondrial function in cardiac cells, reducing susceptibility to treatment-related stress.

Autonomic Regulation

Exercise improves autonomic balance, supporting better rhythm control and faster heart-rate recovery.

Metabolic Protection

Exercise reduces fat mass, preserves muscle, improves lipid profiles, and stabilizes blood glucose, reducing strain on the cardiovascular system.

Exercise Priming Before, During, and After Systemic Therapy

Some people worry that exercising close to chemotherapy or other systemic treatments might increase cardiac strain or worsen cardiotoxicity. Research does not support this concern. Exercise performed before, during, or shortly after systemic therapy is safe when appropriately dosed and does not increase cardiotoxicity.

Light to moderate aerobic activity on infusion days improves circulation, autonomic stability, nausea, and fatigue. During HER2-targeted therapy, structured exercise is safe and may improve heart function. High-intensity training should be avoided immediately after anthracycline infusion, but moderate sessions within the therapeutic window are well tolerated.

Prehabilitation, or exercising in the weeks before therapy, improves cardiorespiratory fitness and may reduce treatment-related cardiac dysfunction. A detailed explanation of exercise priming appears in Chapter 14, but it is important to emphasize here that priming does not increase cardiovascular risk and is frequently beneficial.

Exercise Prescription in Cardio-Oncology

Frequency

Aim for three to five aerobic sessions per week, and two to three resistance sessions on non-consecutive days.

Intensity

Moderate intensity is preferred, corresponding to 60–70% of heart-rate reserve or an effort rating of 4–6 out of 10. Vigorous intervals may be added gradually if tolerated.

Duration

Begin with 20–30 minutes of activity and progress to 40–45 minutes. Shorter bouts are effective on low-energy days.

Mode

Use rhythmic activities involving large muscle groups, such as walking, cycling, swimming, rowing, or stepping. Include resistance training to maintain muscle and bone strength.

Progression

Increase duration first, then intensity, then frequency.

Monitoring and Safety

Heart Rate

Heart-rate monitors help maintain appropriate zones. If taking medications that blunt heart rate, rely more on perceived exertion.

Blood Pressure

Check before and after some sessions, especially when starting new medications. Mild rises during exercise are normal; persistent elevation requires review.

Symptoms Requiring Caution

Stop exercise and seek advice for chest pressure, unusual breathlessness, palpitations, dizziness, or ankle swelling.

Recovery

Heart rate should begin to fall within one minute of stopping. Slow recovery may indicate fatigue.

Professional Oversight

Supervised exercise is recommended for individuals with known cardiovascular disease or those receiving cardiotoxic therapies.

Special Considerations

During Anthracycline Therapy

Light to moderate aerobic exercise is well tolerated and helps preserve cardiac function. Avoid high-intensity work immediately after infusion.

During HER2-Targeted Therapy

Moderate aerobic and resistance training are safe during therapy and may help reverse mild declines in heart function.

After Chest Radiation

Start with gentle mobility and aerobic conditioning. Gradually increase endurance while using breathing and posture work to address chest-wall tightness. Initially limit resistance training to regions not irradiated.

During Hormone Therapy

Combine aerobic and resistance training to counter metabolic and body-composition changes. If bone health permits, include impact work.

Existing Heart Disease

Exercise remains beneficial but requires individualized supervision.

Beyond the Heart: The Cardiometabolic Connection

Many cancer treatments promote metabolic changes that increase cardiovascular risk. Exercise directly targets every component of this cluster.

Insulin Sensitivity and Glucose Control

Exercise improves insulin sensitivity even after a single session and lowers fasting glucose with regular training.

Blood Pressure and Vascular Health

Aerobic training reduces resting blood pressure and improves arterial elasticity.

Lipid Profile and Fat Distribution

Exercise improves HDL, lowers triglycerides, shifts LDL to less inflammatory forms, and reduces visceral fat.

Anti-Inflammatory Effects

Exercise reduces pro-inflammatory cytokines and increases anti-inflammatory myokines.

Prescription for Metabolic Syndrome

- Train 4–5 days weekly using aerobic and resistance training
- Aim for 150–300 minutes of moderate aerobic work or 75–150 minutes vigorous intensity
- Strength train 2–3 times weekly targeting major muscle groups
- Progress gradually and break up prolonged sitting

Practical Application

During Chemotherapy

A 54-year-old woman receiving anthracycline therapy begins a structured walking program at moderate intensity five days per week. She reduces duration on post-infusion days. Over 12 weeks, fatigue improves, resting heart rate decreases, and cardiac function remains stable.

During Androgen Deprivation Therapy

A 68-year-old man alternates aerobic sessions with strength training focused on large compound exercises. Impact training is introduced after 8 weeks of building strength and resilience using heavy resistance training. Blood pressure, lipid profile, glucose, and body composition improve over several months. Bone density is maintained.

Post-Radiation Recovery

A 60-year-old individual recovering from chest radiation starts with seated cycling and breathing exercises, progressing to outdoor walking. Cardiopulmonary endurance improves without worsening chest-wall tightness.

Key Takeaways

- Cancer therapies influence heart and circulatory health, but exercise reduces most risks.
- Aerobic and resistance training improve heart strength, vascular function, blood pressure, metabolic health, and cardiorespiratory fitness.
- Cardiorespiratory fitness strongly predicts long-term survival, and exercise is the most effective way to improve it.
- Exercise priming before, during, and after systemic therapy is safe and does not increase cardiotoxicity.
- Monitoring improves safety, and supervised programs are recommended when cardiotoxic therapies or heart disease are present.

Exercise is a powerful, safe, and accessible cardioprotective therapy. With consistent training, the heart and circulatory system remain strong and resilient throughout cancer treatment and into survivorship.

CHAPTER 28

The Long Game: Exercise for Lifelong Cancer Survivorship

Cancer treatment may end, but the physiological consequences rarely disappear completely. Survivorship is a long phase of care, and exercise remains one of the most effective ways to protect health, restore confidence, and reduce the risk of recurrence or new chronic disease. In this chapter I explain how exercise supports long-term metabolic, cardiovascular, and musculoskeletal health, and how it helps people maintain energy, strength, and independence as the years progress. The goal is not athletic performance but durable wellbeing—building a body that continues to serve you well long after treatment has finished.

Beyond Treatment: Living in Equilibrium

Finishing treatment is not the end of the cancer journey; it marks the beginning of a new phase. Survivorship is about more than remaining disease-free. It is about living in a steady state where the body, mind, and environment support one another.

My goal in this phase is to help people sustain the internal stability we have worked so hard to build. The same biological systems that respond to exercise during treatment—immune, metabolic, vascular, hormonal, and neural—continue to adapt and strengthen for years afterward. Each session of exercise remains a deliberate dose of therapy. It keeps the internal environment cancer-suppressive and protects against the long-term consequences of treatment.

Survivorship is a long game. The choices made now—how you exercise, eat, rest, and manage stress—shape not only how long you live, but how well you live.

The Late Effects of Therapy

Modern cancer treatments have extended survival for millions of people, but they can leave behind persistent physiological strain. Many survivors feel "well" yet describe fatigue, poor sleep, weight gain, muscle loss, or a gradual sense of physical vulnerability.

Common long-term effects include:

- cardiovascular dysfunction related to chemotherapy or radiation
- loss of bone and muscle from hormone therapy or prolonged inactivity
- increased fat mass, metabolic syndrome and insulin resistance
- persistent neuropathy or joint pain
- cognitive fog or reduced attention

Each of these issues is modifiable through targeted exercise medicine. Aerobic training improves vascular health and oxygen delivery. Resistance and impact training rebuild bone and muscle. Interval work improves insulin sensitivity and body composition. Balance and agility drills restore confidence and functional competence. Even cognitive function responds through increases in brain-derived growth factors that support clarity and focus.

The body is continually remodeling. Exercise ensures that this remodeling moves in the right direction.

Exercise as the Foundation of Longevity

For survivors, longevity is not only about preventing recurrence. It is about reducing the risk of the chronic diseases that commonly emerge years after treatment—heart disease, stroke, diabetes, osteoporosis, sarcopenia, and frailty. Exercise is the only single therapy shown to lower risk across all of these conditions.

When performed consistently, exercise:

- lowers inflammation and oxidative stress
- improves lipid and glucose metabolism
- enhances endothelial function and arterial elasticity
- strengthens immune regulation

- supports hormonal stability and circadian rhythm
- improves cognitive performance and emotional resilience

Every one of these mechanisms contributes to maintaining a cancer-suppressive internal environment. In this sense, exercise becomes not only preventive medicine for chronic disease but a long-term maintenance therapy for cancer itself.

The Mindset Shift

In the early stages after treatment, many people still view exercise as something they "should" do. Over time, I aim for them to see it as part of who they are. Physical activity becomes identity—a marker of agency and personal health stewardship.

A major barrier to long-term consistency is the loss of structure. During treatment the calendar is organized around appointments, scans, and cycles. Survivorship removes this external framework, and motivation can fade. Establishing new, meaningful goals restores direction. These goals vary; lifting a grandchild, walking a specific trail, completing a charity ride, or simply regaining a feeling of physical confidence. The aim is not athleticism but ownership of health.

Consistency matters more than intensity. Short, daily episodes of exercise act like maintenance doses of medicine produced by your own physiology. Missing a few days is not failure; it is a signal to gently restore rhythm.

The Evidence for Recurrence Prevention

The evidence supporting exercise for recurrence prevention is compelling. Survivors who maintain regular moderate to vigorous exercise—approximately 150 minutes per week—have substantially lower recurrence and mortality rates across breast, prostate, and colorectal cancers. Risk reductions often fall in the 30–50 percent range!

These effects arise from multiple pathways: improved immune surveillance, reductions in insulin and IGF-1, lower inflammation, healthier body composition, improved cardiovascular function, and more stable tumor biology. Exercise also enhances treatment tolerance, which indirectly influences long-term outcomes.

I often explain to survivors that the most effective long-term "insurance policy" against recurrence is not a supplement or a scan. It is sustained physical activity.

Building a Sustainable Routine

A survivorship plan integrates five essential pillars:

1. **Resistance Training:** Two to four sessions per week targeting all major muscle groups. This preserves lean mass, bone density, and metabolic rate.
2. **Aerobic Conditioning:** At least 150 minutes per week of moderate effort or 75 minutes vigorous effort, accumulated however life allows.
3. **Flexibility and Balance:** Daily short sessions of stretching, yoga, or stability work to maintain mobility and reduce falls risk.
4. **Recovery:** Adequate sleep, hydration, and stress management. Recovery is where adaptations are consolidated.
5. **Purpose:** A clear reason to maintain exercise—health, family, recreation, or service. Purpose sustains the habit when motivation fluctuates.

Programs evolve with age, but the principle remains: keep the heart conditioned, muscles strong, and the mind engaged.

The Power of Small Actions

Many survivors believe they need dramatic changes to maintain their health. They do not. The body responds to every positive signal. A ten-minute walk after meals smooths post-meal glucose spikes. Small daily sets of squats or step-ups preserve leg strength and independence. A short resistance session twice weekly slows bone and muscle loss. These modest actions accumulate into profound long-term benefit.

The secret to survivorship is not dramatic effort but steady persistence. The body rewards consistency with resilience.

Closing Reflections

Cancer forces people to confront mortality, but it also provides an opportunity to live with greater intention. Survivorship is not merely the absence of disease; it is the presence of vitality, autonomy, and steady physical capability.

Exercise medicine is the foundation of this vitality. It converts uncertainty into action and strengthens the physiological systems that support long-term wellbeing. My aim is to help every survivor not only live longer but live better—to wake with energy, move with confidence, and contribute each day to their own recovery.

This is the long game of cancer survivorship: a life shaped not by the memory of disease, but by the presence of strength.

CHAPTER 29

The Path Forward: Living with Strength and Purpose

Reaching the end of treatment or the end of this book is not the end of the cancer journey. It is the beginning of a new phase—one defined not by appointments or scans, but by your daily choices. These choices shape the internal environment of your body far more than most people realize. They influence how you feel, how you function, how you age, and how resilient you remain in the years ahead.

If there is one message I want you to take forward, it is this: exercise is not optional. It is essential. Not because it improves fitness or appearance, but because it is a clinically proven therapy that protects every organ and system cancer touches—heart, muscle, brain, metabolism, immunity, hormones, cognition, and emotional wellbeing.

Exercise is a form of medicine, and with the right guidance you can deliver it safely every day. Some people feel confident following a self-directed plan, while others benefit from partnering with a clinical exercise physiologist, physiotherapist, or trained fitness professional. What matters is that exercise becomes part of your long-term care, tailored to your body, your history, and your goals.

Staying in the Therapeutic Zone

Your body is always adapting. It remodels in response to the signals you give it. When you train regularly, you reinforce strength, vascular health, immune surveillance, metabolic stability, and mental clarity. When you become inactive, the same systems begin to drift. Fatigue accumulates, muscle quality declines, glucose regulation worsens, and inflammation rises.

Survivorship is about staying in the therapeutic zone—small daily doses of activity that keep your physiology aligned with health rather than disease. It does not require heroic effort. It requires consistency.

- A ten-minute walk after meals.
- Two sets of resistance exercises before breakfast.
- A short interval session once or twice a week.
- Impact work to protect bone.
- Stretching and balance work for joint health and confidence.

These are not dramatic actions. They are steady signals that tell your body what you expect from it.

Exercise as an Ongoing Partnership

No matter your age, diagnosis, or treatment history, the benefits of exercise accumulate. You are not competing with anyone. You are shaping your own biology, one session at a time.

I have worked with survivors in their twenties and others in their nineties. I have seen people recover from years of deconditioning, rebuild muscle despite hormone therapy, regain balance after neuropathy, re-establish their identity after fatigue, and reconnect with their bodies after surgery. None of this happens overnight. All of it happens through repeated small steps.

View exercise as a partnership between you and your physiology. Clinical treatments target the disease; exercise shapes the environment in which the disease exists. Together, they form a more complete model of care.

Protecting Your Future Health

For many people, cancer increases the risk of other chronic conditions—heart disease, diabetes, osteoporosis, sarcopenia, and frailty. These are not inevitable. Exercise reduces the risk of each of them while also lowering the likelihood of cancer recurrence. There is no drug, procedure, or supplement that matches this spectrum of benefit.

Your goal now is long-term healthspan—the number of years lived with strength, clarity, mobility, and independence. Exercise is the foundation of that healthspan. Its benefits compound over time.

Purpose Beyond Treatment

After treatment ends, structure disappears, and many survivors feel adrift. Setting new goals restores direction. These goals do not need to be athletic. They need to be meaningful: being able to travel, return to a hobby, play with grandchildren, sleep more soundly, reduce reliance on medications, or simply regain a sense of physical confidence.

Purpose sustains habit when motivation fades. Purpose will carry you further than willpower.

Your Agency Matters

Cancer removes many choices. Exercise gives some of them back. Every session is a reminder that you can influence your internal environment, stabilize what treatment disrupted, and build resilience for the future.

Your body remains responsive. It adapts, strengthens, and improves. No matter how much treatment has challenged you, there is always room to rebuild.

The path forward is not defined by the absence of disease but by the presence of vitality. Exercise medicine is the foundation of this vitality. It converts uncertainty into action and strengthens the physiological systems that support long-term wellbeing.

My aim is to help every survivor not only live longer but live better—to wake with energy, move with confidence, and contribute each day to their own recovery.

This is the long game of cancer survivorship: a life shaped not by the memory of disease, but by the presence of strength.

And whether you continue independently or with the support of qualified professionals, exercise remains the most reliable tool you have to shape your future health—one session at a time.

Epilogue

Exercise Medicine Across the Entire Cancer Journey

Cancer changes a life from the moment of diagnosis, and the need for strength — physical, psychological, and physiological — begins immediately. Throughout this book, I have shown that exercise is not a temporary intervention or an optional add-on. It is a therapy that remains relevant across every phase of cancer care. Before treatment begins, exercise prepares the body and mind for what lies ahead. During chemotherapy, radiation, immunotherapy, surgery, or hormone therapy, it improves treatment tolerance, **increases the safety and effectiveness of all cancer treatments**, reduces side effects, and protects the systems most under stress. After treatment, exercise becomes rehabilitation, restoring the strength, metabolism, and capacity that illness and therapy often erode. In survivorship, it preserves long-term health, reduces recurrence risk, and stabilizes the internal environment. And even in advanced or palliative care, exercise maintains comfort, mobility, and autonomy for as long as possible. The purpose changes, but the value does not.

If there is one message I want you to carry with you, it is this: exercise is always relevant. No matter the cancer type, stage, treatment plan, prognosis, or physical capacity, there is always a form of exercise that can strengthen physiology and support wellbeing.

Exercise is a form of medicine, and with the right guidance you can deliver it safely every day. Some people feel confident following a self-directed plan, while others benefit from partnering with a clinical exercise physiologist, physiotherapist, or trained fitness professional. Both paths are valid. What matters is that exercise becomes a stable part of your care, matched to your condition, symptoms, and goals.

Cancer can alter physiology, function, identity, and daily life, but it does not remove the body's ability to adapt. You now understand the mechanisms behind exercise medicine: how muscle supports immunity, how circulation and oxygenation influence treatment effectiveness, how exercise protects the heart, brain, and metabolism, and how small, regular sessions shift the internal environment toward health.

With this knowledge comes agency. At any stage of the cancer journey — newly diagnosed, mid-treatment, recovering, living with advanced disease, or supporting someone you love — exercise offers a way to participate actively in your own care. This does not require dramatic goals. It requires rhythm and repetition: the accumulated benefit of daily choices rather than occasional effort.

Survivorship is sometimes portrayed as a return to normality, but in reality it is an evolution into a new phase of life — one shaped by purposeful actions rather than passive waiting. Exercise helps define that phase. It supports a physiology capable of healing, stabilizing, and enduring.

My aim in writing this book was to give you the understanding, confidence, and clarity to use exercise as medicine at every stage of the journey. Whether your goal is to tolerate treatment better, rebuild strength, protect long-term health, maintain independence, or support comfort and dignity, exercise provides a path forward grounded in evidence and guided by your own capacity.

Cancer may change the future you expected, but it does not remove your influence over the future you can build. Exercise medicine gives you a way to shape that future — with intention, knowledge, and persistence — one carefully chosen session at a time.

And whether you continue independently or with the support of qualified professionals, exercise remains the most reliable tool you have to support your physiology and strengthen your resilience across the entire cancer journey.

About the Author

Professor Robert U. Newton, BHMS(Hons), MHMS, PhD, DSc, AEP, FAHMS, FESSA, FACSM, FNSCA

Professor Robert Newton is an internationally recognised leader in exercise oncology and one of the world's most published researchers on exercise as medicine for cancer. He is Professor of Exercise Medicine at Edith Cowan University in Perth, Western Australia, where he established the Exercise Medicine Research Institute—one of the first centres globally dedicated to the scientific study of exercise as a therapeutic modality in oncology.

Across a career spanning more than four decades, Professor Newton has conducted pioneering research on how targeted exercise can improve treatment tolerance, influence tumour biology, and preserve muscle, bone, and metabolic health during and after cancer therapy. His work has helped define exercise medicine as neoadjuvant, adjuvant, and rehabilitative therapy in cancer care and has shaped clinical guidelines internationally.

He has authored more than **1,000 scientific publications**, including **587 peer-reviewed journal articles**, **19 book chapters**, and several books. His research has been cited more than **37,000 times**, with an h-index of 102—placing him among the most influential scientists in the field. He has attracted more than **$51 million in competitive research funding** across 161 grants, including major awards from the NHMRC, Cancer Australia, the Movember Foundation, and the World Cancer Research Fund.

Professor Newton holds fellowships in the **Australian Academy of Health and Medical Sciences**, the **American College of Sports Medicine, Exercise and Sports Science Australia**, and the **National Strength and Conditioning Association**. He is an Accredited Exercise Physiologist, Certified Strength and Conditioning Specialist, and a member of key national and international oncology organisations including the Clinical Oncology Society of Australia and the American Society of Clinical Oncology.

His scientific leadership has been recognised through major awards, including **Western Australia Premier's Scientist of the Year (2019)**, the Cancer Council WA **Research Career Achievement Award (2018)**, and numerous national and international honours. In 2021, The University of Queensland awarded him the degree of Doctor of Science for his lifetime contribution to exercise oncology.

Professor Newton has supervised more than **80 doctoral and master's graduates**, many of whom are now research and clinical leaders in oncology worldwide. His research teams collaborate internationally across hospitals, cancer centres, universities, and clinical trials groups to advance precision exercise medicine and integrative cancer care.

MyExerciseMedicine for Cancer brings together Professor Newton's personal experience, scientific discoveries, and decades of clinical practice to provide patients, survivors, families, and clinicians with a clear, evidence-based path to using exercise as a safe and powerful treatment.

Glossary

A

Absolute Contraindication – A situation where exercise must not be performed due to high risk (e.g., unstable angina, severe anemia).

Active Surveillance – Monitoring certain cancers without immediate treatment, using PSA, imaging, or biopsies.

Adjuvant Exercise Medicine – Exercise performed during active cancer treatment to improve tolerance, reduce toxicity, and enhance effectiveness.

Adjuvant Therapy – Treatment given after primary therapy (e.g., after surgery) to reduce recurrence.

Aerobic Capacity – The ability of the heart, lungs, and muscles to take in, deliver, and use oxygen during exercise.

Aerobic Exercise – Continuous rhythmic exercise (walking, cycling, swimming) that raises heart rate and breathing.

Aging-Related Muscle Loss (Sarcopenia) – Decline in muscle quantity and quality with aging; accelerated by cancer treatment.

AIs (Aromatase Inhibitors) – Breast cancer hormone therapy drugs that reduce estrogen.

Aldosterone – Hormone influencing fluid balance; affected by exercise and medications.

Anaerobic Threshold – The exercise intensity at which lactate begins to accumulate; useful for setting training zones.

Anabolic Resistance – Reduced ability to build muscle, common in cachexia and aging.

Androgen Deprivation Therapy (ADT) – Hormone therapy for prostate cancer that lowers testosterone.

Angiogenesis – Formation of new blood vessels; exercise normalises tumour vasculature.

Anabolic Signalling – Biological signals that stimulate muscle growth; activated by resistance training.

Antiemetic – Medication that reduces nausea.

Anti-inflammatory Myokines – Molecules released by muscle during exercise that reduce inflammation.

Autonomic Nervous System (ANS) – Regulates stress response, heart rate, digestion, and sleep; exercise improves balance.

B

BCAAs (Branched-Chain Amino Acids) – Leucine, isoleucine, valine—important for muscle repair.

BDNF (Brain-Derived Neurotrophic Factor) – A protein that supports brain health, learning, mood; increased by exercise.

Behavioral Activation – Psychological strategy using action to influence mood; exercise is a core example.

Bioimpedance Spectroscopy (BIS) – Technology to detect early lymphedema.

Biological Age – A measure of physiological aging vs chronological age.

Biomechanics – Study of how the body moves; essential for safe exercise technique.

Biotherapy – Cancer treatment using biological agents.

Blood–Brain Barrier – Protective barrier around the brain that can be affected by treatment.

Blood Glucose Variability – Fluctuations in glucose; stabilised by exercise.

Bone Mineral Density (BMD) – Measurement of bone strength via DEXA.

Breath-Hold (DIBH) – Technique used in left-sided breast radiation to reduce cardiac exposure.

Burst Exercise – Short intensifications used in interval training.

C

Cachexia – A complex metabolic syndrome causing muscle loss and weight decline in cancer.

Cancer-Suppressive Environment – A physiological state promoted by exercise, characterised by low inflammation, stable metabolism, and strong immunity.

Cardio-Metabolic Health – Combined cardiovascular and metabolic function; improved with exercise.

Cardio-Oncology – The field that examines how cancer and treatments affect the heart.

Cardiorespiratory Fitness (CRF) – The strongest predictor of survival in many cancers.

CAR-T Therapy – Cell-based immunotherapy using genetically modified T-cells.

Catabolic State – A breakdown state where muscle loss exceeds repair.

CEPs (Clinical Exercise Physiologists) – Allied health professionals trained to prescribe exercise as medical therapy.

Chemobrain / CRCI – Cancer-related cognitive impairment.

Chemoradiation – Combined chemotherapy and radiation therapy.

CIPN (Chemotherapy-Induced Peripheral Neuropathy) – Nerve damage from treatment.

Circadian Rhythm – The body's 24-hour physiological cycle; exercise and light entrain it.

Compression Garments – Medical garments used in lymphedema.

Concentric Contraction – Muscle shortening during lifting.

Cortisol – Stress hormone elevated during illness and poor sleep; stabilised by exercise.

CTDNA (Circulating Tumor DNA) – Tumour fragments detected in blood.

Cytokines – Immune signalling molecules; some are inflammatory, some anti-inflammatory.

D

Delayed-Onset Muscle Soreness (DOMS) – Soreness after new or intense exercise; reduced by gradual progression.

DEXA Scan – Measures lean mass, fat mass, and bone density.

DNA Repair – Cellular mechanisms that fix damage; enhanced by exercise.

Dose–Response (Exercise) – Relationship where more consistent exercise yields more benefit.

Drop Set – Resistance-training technique to increase metabolic stress.

Dyspnea – Shortness of breath.

E

Energy Flux – Relationship between energy intake and expenditure.

Endocrine Therapy – Hormone treatment for breast or prostate cancer.

Endothelium – Lining of blood vessels; becomes healthier with exercise.

EPOC (Excess Post-Exercise Oxygen Consumption) – "Afterburn" where metabolism remains elevated after training.

Exergaming – Exercise combined with virtual or digital platforms.

Exercise Medicine – The clinical use of exercise as a therapeutic intervention.

Exercise Priming – Targeted exercise before, during, or after treatment to enhance therapy effectiveness.

Exercise Snacks – Short, frequent bouts of movement to reduce sedentary time.

Exercise Tolerance – Ability to withstand exercise without adverse effect.

F

Fatigue (Cancer-Related) – Persistent exhaustion not relieved by rest; exercise is the best treatment.

FITT-VP – Framework for prescribing exercise: Frequency, Intensity, Time, Type, Volume, Progression.

Flow Cytometry – Lab technique to analyse immune cells.

Functional Capacity – Ability to perform daily tasks; strongly influenced by exercise.

G

Glycemic Control – Regulation of blood sugar; improved by resistance and aerobic exercise.

Glycogen – Stored carbohydrate in liver and muscle.

Grade Group (Prostate Cancer) – Modern replacement for Gleason scoring.

Growth Factors – Biological signals controlling cell growth; modulated by exercise.

Gut Microbiome – Intestinal microbial ecosystem influenced by exercise and diet.

H

Hb (Hemoglobin) – Protein in red blood cells that carries oxygen.

Heart-Rate Reserve (HRR) – HRmax – resting HR; basis for the Karvonen formula.

Heat Shock Proteins (HSPs) – Protective proteins increased by exercise.

HITT / HIIT – High-intensity interval training.

Hormesis – Beneficial adaptation arising from small, controlled stress (e.g., exercise).

Hypoxia – Low oxygen; exercise reduces tumour hypoxia.

I

Immune Checkpoint Inhibitors – Immunotherapy drugs that reactivate T-cells.

Immune Surveillance – The immune system's ability to detect abnormal cells; enhanced by exercise.

Inflammation (Chronic) – Persistent immune activation; countered by exercise.

Insulin Resistance – Reduced ability of cells to respond to insulin.

Interval Training – Alternating effort and recovery.

Isometric Exercise – Holding tension without movement.

J–K

Joint Effusion – Fluid around a joint.

Karvonen Formula – Method for prescribing heart-rate training zones.

L

Lean Mass – Muscle, bone, organs; protected by resistance training.

Left Ventricular Ejection Fraction (LVEF) – Measure of heart pumping.

Leukapheresis – Cell collection for CAR-T therapy.

Lymphedema – Swelling from impaired lymphatic drainage; exercise is safe and beneficial.

Lymphangion – Contractile segment of a lymph vessel.

M

Maximal Aerobic Power – VO_2max; peak oxygen uptake.

Mediterranean Diet – Plant-forward eating pattern supporting metabolic and cardiovascular health.

Metabolic Flexibility – Ability to switch between fuel sources efficiently.

Metabolic Syndrome – Cluster of metabolic abnormalities; reduced by exercise.

Mitochondria – Cell energy factories; increased by exercise.

Mixed-Mode Training – Combining aerobic and resistance work.

Moderate Intensity – Exercise at RPE 4–6 or talk-but-not-sing level.

Muscle Hypertrophy – Increase in muscle size.

Myokines – Beneficial molecules released from contracting muscle.

N

Neoadjuvant Exercise – Exercise before treatment (prehabilitation).

Neutropenia – Low neutrophils; infection risk.

Neuromuscular Coordination – Control of movement patterns.

Non-Exercise Activity Thermogenesis (NEAT) – Energy expended outside formal exercise.

O

Oncology Rehabilitation – Exercise-led recovery during and after treatment.

Oxidative Stress – Imbalance of free radicals; exercise strengthens antioxidant defences.

Overload Principle – Increasing challenge to stimulate adaptation.

P

Palliative Exercise – Exercise to maintain comfort and function in advanced disease.

Peak VO_2 – Highest oxygen uptake; critical fitness measure.

Pelvic-Floor Strength – Supports continence and sexual function.

Peripheral Neuropathy – Nerve dysfunction; improved with exercise.

Periodization – Planned sequencing of training loads.

Platelet Count – Blood-clotting measure relevant for exercise safety.

Precision Exercise Oncology – Tailoring exercise to tumour biology, treatment stage, and physiology.

Protein Synthesis – Building muscle; stimulated by resistance training.

Psychophysiology – Interaction between mind and body; influenced by exercise.

Q

Quality of Life (QoL) – Overall wellbeing; consistently improved by exercise.

R

RPE (Rating of Perceived Exertion) – 0–10 scale for subjective exercise intensity.

Recovery – Physiological rebuilding after exercise; includes sleep, nutrition, active rest.

Resistance Training – Exercises using load to build strength and muscle.

Resting Metabolic Rate (RMR) – Baseline calorie burn.

ROM (Range of Motion) – Joint mobility.

S

Sedentary Behaviour – Prolonged sitting; harmful independent of exercise.

Self-Efficacy – Belief in one's ability to act; strengthened by successful exercise.

Sentinel Node – First node draining a tumour area.

Sleep Architecture – Pattern of REM and non-REM sleep.

Stress Hormones – Cortisol, adrenaline; regulated by exercise.

Strength Curve – Force capacity across joint angles.

Survivorship – The long-term phase of life after treatment.

T

Talk Test – Simple measure of intensity: can talk = moderate; short phrases = vigorous.

T-Cell Exhaustion – Loss of immune effectiveness; exercise reverses aspects of this.

Therapeutic Window (Exercise) – Optimal timing around cancer treatment to enhance effect.

Theranostics – Combined diagnostic-imaging and targeted radiotherapy.

TNM Staging – Tumour size (T), lymph nodes (N), metastases (M).

Tumour Microenvironment – Biological ecosystem surrounding cancer cells; modified by exercise.

U–Z

VO_2peak – Peak aerobic capacity.

Vascular Elasticity – Vessel flexibility; improved with training.

Wearables – Devices that track HR, sleep, steps, and intensity; useful for autoregulation.

Zone Training – Exercise performed in specific heart-rate or RPE zones.

APPENDIX A

Cancer Biology, Diagnosis, and Treatment: A Practical Reference

Introduction

This appendix provides a factual overview of cancer biology, global incidence, the principles behind diagnosis, the tests used to confirm cancer, and the foundational concepts that shape treatment decisions. It is intended as a clear reference you can return to at any time — whether you are newly diagnosed, supporting someone through treatment, or wanting to understand the medical language used throughout oncology. The focus here is clarity and accuracy rather than emotion. Understanding this framework makes the rest of the book easier to interpret.

What Exactly Is Cancer?

Cancer begins when normal cells lose the controls that regulate their growth and behavior. In the body's usual system, each cell follows a disciplined cycle: it divides only when needed, checks its DNA for errors at specific checkpoints, repairs mistakes when possible, and undergoes programed cell death (apoptosis) when damaged or no longer required. These safeguards keep tissues healthy and prevent uncontrolled growth.

A cell becomes cancerous when several of these safeguards fail. It may stop repairing DNA properly, override the internal signals that normally prevent excessive division, ignore instructions to self-destruct, or develop the ability to escape the boundaries of the tissue where it began. Two cancers that look similar under a microscope can behave very differently depending on which cellular safeguards were lost first, which mutations accumulated later, and how the surrounding environment interacts with the tumor.

The process is seldom triggered by a single cause. Most cancers follow a **multiple-hit model**, in which several small defects accumulate over many years. Some of these defects arise from the normal aging process; others are influenced by environmental exposures such as ultraviolet radiation, tobacco smoke, air pollution, occupational chemicals, chronic inflammation, or infections like HPV, hepatitis B and C, or Helicobacter pylori. A smaller proportion of cancers arise partly from inherited genetic variants that predispose someone to higher risk, though even in these cases, additional changes usually need to occur before cancer develops.

Benign versus malignant tumors

Not all abnormal growths are cancer. *Benign tumors* can enlarge and cause symptoms by pressing on nearby structures, but they do not invade or spread. *Malignant tumors* can invade neighboring tissues and may spread through lymphatic channels or blood vessels.

When malignant cells travel to distant sites — a process called *metastasis* — they retain the characteristics of their original tissue. For example, cancer that begins in the colon but spreads to the liver remains colon cancer and is treated according to colon cancer biology. The site of spread changes the prognosis and treatment strategy, but the cancer's identity stays the same.

Cancer by the Numbers

Cancer is common worldwide. In 2022, approximately **20 million** people were newly diagnosed and just under **10 million** died from cancer-related causes. These numbers continue to rise as populations grow and age, and because many risk factors — including tobacco use, alcohol consumption, obesity, and air pollution — remain widespread. Forecasts suggest that global cancer incidence may reach **around 35 million cases per year** by mid-century.

Patterns differ across countries and between sexes. Breast cancer remains the most common cancer diagnosed in women worldwide. Lung cancer is a leading diagnosis in many countries and the leading cause of cancer death overall. In men, prostate cancer and lung cancer are the most common. Colorectal cancer affects both sexes and is influenced by lifestyle, diet, genetics, and participation in screening programs.

Why do statistics vary so widely between regions? Differences in lifestyle exposures, genetics, vaccination programs, environmental conditions, and healthcare access all play a role. Countries with strong screening programs and timely access to treatment typically diagnose cancers earlier — when they are most treatable — and achieve better long-term outcomes.

Interpreting statistics

Statistics are helpful for understanding public health trends, but they do not predict what will happen to any individual.

- **Incidence** describes how many people are diagnosed.
- **Mortality** describes how many die from cancer.
- **Survival rates** describe outcomes in past patient groups; they cannot forecast an individual outcome and often lag behind current treatment advances.

For individuals, prognosis depends on the **type, stage, molecular features**, and the **quality and availability of treatment**, as well as general health and access to supportive care. Population averages offer context, not destiny.

The Principles Behind Good Testing

Cancer diagnosis relies on structured, evidence-based pathways. Every test serves a purpose and helps answer a specific clinical question.

Screening tests aim to detect abnormalities when cancer is small or before symptoms appear. They are not designed to diagnose cancer — only to identify who should undergo more definitive tests.

To confirm a diagnosis, tissue is required. A biopsy provides this tissue, enabling a pathologist to examine the cells directly. Once cancer is confirmed, imaging determines where it is, how large it has grown, whether nearby lymph nodes are involved, and whether there is spread to other organs. Further laboratory, molecular, or genomic tests refine the understanding of the tumor and guide modern treatment selection.

Sensitivity and specificity

No test is perfect.

- **Sensitivity** measures how often a test correctly identifies cancer when it is present.
- **Specificity** measures how often a test correctly identifies the absence of cancer when it is not present.

A highly sensitive test catches most cases but may produce more false positives. A highly specific test reduces false alarms but may miss early disease. That is why testing follows a layered approach: **screen → confirm → stage → characterize**. Each step builds confidence and reduces uncertainty.

False positives can lead to unnecessary worry and additional testing. False negatives can give false reassurance. Understanding these limitations helps explain why clinicians choose certain pathways and why multiple tests are often required.

From Concern to Confirmation: Biopsies and Cytology

A biopsy is the most definitive way to diagnose cancer. Imaging can strongly suggest cancer, but only a tissue or cell sample can confirm it.

Biopsies are performed using different techniques depending on the location, size, accessibility, and nature of the abnormality. The goal is always the same: obtain enough tissue to make an accurate diagnosis with minimal risk to the patient.

Fine-needle aspiration (FNA)

Uses a very thin needle to draw out cells. It is quick, usually well-tolerated, and ideal for superficial nodes, thyroid nodules, or cystic structures.

Core needle biopsy

Removes small cores of tissue. Because it preserves the architecture of the tissue, it is essential for diagnosing many tumors such as breast, prostate, or soft-tissue lesions.

Vacuum-assisted biopsy

Uses a powered device to obtain multiple cores through a single entry point. It is particularly useful in breast imaging when a larger sample is needed.

Incisional and excisional biopsies

A surgeon may remove part of a lesion (incisional) or the entire lesion (excisional) when needle methods cannot provide adequate information.

Bone marrow aspiration and trephine biopsy

These procedures sample the blood-forming tissue and are central to diagnosing leukemias, lymphomas, myeloma, and unexplained blood abnormalities.

Sentinel lymph node biopsy

Used in breast cancer, melanoma, and other cancers to identify the first lymph node(s) draining the tumor region. If these nodes are free of cancer, further node removal may not be required.

Endoscopic and bronchoscopic biopsies

Endoscopic ultrasound allows sampling of structures behind the stomach or near the pancreas. Bronchoscopy with EBUS enables sampling of masses or lymph nodes in the chest.

Image-guided biopsy

Ultrasound, CT, or MRI is often used to guide the needle into deeper or smaller lesions with accuracy and safety.

What the Pathologist Looks For

The pathology report is the cancer's identity document. It confirms whether cancer is present, identifies the type, and provides crucial details about its behavior.

Pathologists examine:

- **Cell morphology and architecture**, which determine the tumor's classification and **grade**.
- **Immunohistochemistry (IHC)**, which detects proteins expressed by the tumor. These may indicate how the tumor

grows and which therapies may work (e.g., hormone receptors and HER2 in breast cancer; PD-L1 in several cancers; mismatch-repair proteins in colorectal cancer).

- **Molecular and genomic characteristics**, including mutations, gene fusions, or structural changes detected by next-generation sequencing, PCR, or FISH. These findings guide targeted therapies such as EGFR or ALK inhibitors in lung cancer, BRAF inhibitors in melanoma, or PARP inhibitors in BRCA-related cancers.
- **Blood cancer markers**, using flow cytometry and cytogenetics to classify leukemias and lymphomas and identify specific translocations such as BCR-ABL1.

This level of detail increasingly shapes treatment decisions. Oncology has shifted from treating tumors solely by location to treating them according to their **biology and molecular drivers**, making pathology essential in modern cancer care.

Imaging: Mapping the Territory

Imaging is central to modern cancer care. It helps locate tumors, measure them, understand their relationship with surrounding structures, guide biopsies, plan treatment, and monitor response. Each imaging modality has strengths, limitations, and ideal uses.

X-rays remain a simple starting point for certain situations. They provide quick views of bones and the chest and can detect fractures, lung abnormalities, or obvious masses. Their simplicity is useful, but they lack the detail needed for deeper or smaller lesions.

Ultrasound uses sound waves to generate images of soft tissues. It is accessible, free of radiation, and excellent for guiding biopsies of the thyroid, breast, lymph nodes, and abdominal organs. It is operator-dependent, but in experienced hands it is invaluable.

CT (computed tomography) produces detailed cross-sectional images and is a cornerstone of cancer staging. CT scans show organ structure, lymph nodes, and potential metastatic sites. Intravenous contrast enhances detail but requires attention to kidney function and possible allergies.

MRI provides superior soft-tissue contrast without radiation. It is particularly useful for the brain and spinal cord, liver, pelvis, and musculoskeletal tumors. MRI sequences can distinguish subtle tissue differences far better than CT. Some metal implants and specific devices are incompatible with MRI, and gadolinium contrast is used selectively based on renal function and diagnostic need.

PET/CT and PET/MRI offer metabolic imaging by combining an anatomical scan with a tracer that highlights active or abnormal cells. The most common tracer is FDG, a glucose analogue, which is taken up by many cancers. Some tumor types require specialized tracers such as PSMA for prostate cancer or DOTATATE for neuroendocrine tumors. PET imaging is powerful for staging, planning, and assessing treatment response.

Nuclear medicine bone scans detect areas of increased bone turnover and are commonly used in cancers that tend to spread to bone, such as prostate and breast cancer.

For liver lesions, **contrast-enhanced ultrasound**, **multiphase CT**, and **multiphase MRI** help distinguish benign from malignant patterns. In people with cirrhosis, certain characteristic imaging patterns allow hepatocellular carcinoma to be diagnosed without biopsy.

Across all modalities, clinicians balance the diagnostic value of an imaging test with safety considerations such as radiation exposure, kidney function, the need for sedation, and potential contrast reactions.

Endoscopy and Minimally Invasive Scopes

Endoscopic procedures allow clinicians to visualize internal surfaces directly and perform targeted biopsies or treatments.

Colonoscopy examines the lining of the large bowel and is used both to investigate symptoms and to follow up positive stool-based screening tests. It can detect and remove polyps, some of which are pre-cancerous. **Flexible sigmoidoscopy** views the lower colon only and is used in selected screening programs.

Upper endoscopy (gastroscopy) visualizes the esophagus, stomach, and duodenum. It can detect inflammation, ulcers, strictures, and early cancers, and it allows biopsies to be taken during the same procedure.

Bronchoscopy examines the airways and can sample lung masses or lymph nodes in the chest. When paired with endobronchial ultrasound (EBUS), it becomes a precise tool for staging lung cancer.

Cystoscopy views the bladder lining and is essential for diagnosing and monitoring bladder cancer. Because many bladder cancers recur, cystoscopy is often part of long-term follow-up.

Hysteroscopy and colposcopy allow direct examination of the uterus and cervix. These tests are typically performed after abnormal Pap or HPV results or in response to abnormal bleeding.

ERCP and **MRCP** evaluate the bile ducts and pancreas when blockages or strictures are suspected. **Endoscopic ultrasound (EUS)** adds detailed imaging from within the gastrointestinal tract and allows biopsies of deep structures.

Capsule endoscopy involves swallowing a small camera that transmits images of the small intestine, which cannot be reached by standard endoscopy. It is useful when other investigations are inconclusive.

Blood Tests and Tumor Markers

Routine blood tests evaluate blood counts, liver and kidney function, electrolytes, inflammation, and metabolic status. They provide a broad understanding of overall health and help determine whether it is safe to proceed with treatments such as surgery, chemotherapy, or immunotherapy.

Tumor markers are substances—usually proteins—that may be elevated in the blood of some people with certain cancers. They are not reliable for general cancer screening, as many benign conditions can elevate them and many cancers do not produce markers at early stages.

Markers include PSA (prostate cancer), CA-125 (ovarian cancer), CEA (colon cancer), CA 19-9 (pancreatic cancer), AFP (primary liver cancer and some germ-cell tumors), hCG (germ-cell tumors), calcitonin (medullary thyroid cancer), and chromogranin A (some neuroendocrine tumors). In practice, tumor markers are primarily used to assess treatment response and monitor for recurrence, not to detect cancer in the first place.

Because many factors influence marker levels, changes are interpreted in context, and isolated abnormalities rarely drive major decisions without supporting evidence.

Liquid Biopsy and Circulating Tumor DNA (ctDNA)

Liquid biopsy refers to analyzing cancer-related genetic material circulating in the bloodstream. It has two main uses.

First, it can help identify actionable mutations when tissue biopsy is difficult, risky, or insufficient. This is most relevant when cancers evolve over time and develop new mutations that may respond to targeted therapies.

Second, liquid biopsies can detect minimal residual disease (MRD) after treatment. MRD refers to tiny amounts of cancer that remain after surgery or chemotherapy—levels too low to see on scans. Measuring ctDNA can sometimes identify recurrence risk earlier than imaging.

The field is advancing quickly. While liquid biopsy is extremely promising, particularly for MRD detection, how best to use the information varies by cancer type. It does not replace tissue diagnosis but can complement it at key decision points.

Screening Tests and Follow-Up Pathways

Screening aims to detect cancers or pre-cancerous changes before symptoms appear. Effective screening programs reduce mortality by finding disease earlier, when treatment is more likely to be successful. The specific approach depends on the cancer type, the population, and local guidelines.

Breast cancer screening commonly uses mammography, sometimes with added ultrasound or MRI in higher-risk groups. **Bowel cancer screening** often begins with stool-based tests such as FIT or FOBT, followed by colonoscopy if positive.

Cervical cancer screening relies on HPV-based testing and, when abnormal, colposcopy and biopsy. **Lung cancer screening** with low-dose CT is recommended for some current and former smokers at higher risk.

A positive screening test does not diagnose cancer. It indicates the need for confirmatory imaging or biopsy. Well-designed programs explain next steps, help manage anxiety, and avoid unnecessary delays.

When the Diagnosis Is Complex

Some cancers require specialized pathways because of their anatomy, biology, or behavior.

- **Melanoma** is best diagnosed with complete excision of the suspicious mole whenever possible. Depth of invasion (Breslow thickness) determines the need for sentinel node biopsy.
- **Sarcoma** evaluation begins with imaging and requires a biopsy performed along a path that can be removed during surgery. MRI plays a central role.
- **Pancreatic cancer** often requires multiphase CT or MRI combined with EUS-guided biopsy; CA 19-9 is used as an adjunct.
- **Hepatocellular carcinoma** in cirrhosis can sometimes be diagnosed based on characteristic imaging features alone.
- **Thyroid nodules** are assessed with high-resolution ultrasound and fine-needle aspiration; molecular classifiers assist when results are indeterminate.
- **Blood cancers** require a combination of blood tests, peripheral smear analysis, bone marrow biopsy, flow cytometry, and genetic testing.
- **Prostate cancer** uses PSA and MRI to guide targeted transperineal biopsies. PSMA PET is becoming increasingly important for staging.

- **Neuroendocrine tumors** may require DOTATATE PET/CT, chromogranin A testing, or 24-hour urine 5-HIAA depending on the subtype.
- **Brain tumors** are primarily assessed with MRI, followed by surgery aimed at maximal safe resection and tissue diagnosis.

Accurate diagnosis relies on choosing the right tests in the correct sequence.

Preparing for Tests: Practical Notes

Different tests have different preparation requirements, and following them improves safety and accuracy.

- Always inform your team of allergies, especially to iodinated contrast.
- Tell your clinicians about kidney problems, pacemakers, implants, pregnancy, or the possibility of pregnancy.
- Some scans require fasting; others require drinking water or contrast.
- For procedures with sedation (such as colonoscopy or some biopsies), arrange a driver.
- Bring previous imaging or ensure the imaging center can access older scans for comparison.
- If you are on blood thinners, ask whether they should be paused before a biopsy or endoscopy.

Small steps can prevent complications and ensure the smoothest possible process.

Staging: Creating a Map

Staging describes the extent of cancer and helps guide treatment planning. The **TNM system** is the most widely used.

- **T** describes the size or depth of the primary tumor.
- **N** describes whether nearby lymph nodes are involved.

- **M** indicates whether there is distant metastasis.

These details are grouped into **Stages 0–IV**:

- **Stage 0** involves very early disease limited to the surface layer of tissue.
- **Stage I** is small and confined to its site of origin.
- **Stage II** is larger or has grown more deeply.
- **Stage III** involves lymph nodes or local extension into nearby structures.
- **Stage IV** indicates spread to distant organs or tissues.

The same stage number can mean different things in different cancers, and biology often modifies stage-based decisions. Some aggressive tumors behave more like higher-stage disease; some slow-growing tumors behave more indolently even when advanced.

Staging allows clinicians to compare outcomes, plan treatment, and communicate clearly across teams.

Prostate Cancer Explained: The Gleason Score and Grade Groups

Prostate cancer grading is unique and often confusing to patients. The most common grading system is the **Gleason score**, which identifies patterns in the cancer cells and adds the two most common patterns together. Each pattern is graded from 3 to 5, and the sum becomes the Gleason score (from 6 to 10). This is then translated into **Grade Groups**, which simplify risk discussions.

- **Grade Group 1**: Gleason 6 (3+3) — lower-grade, often suitable for active surveillance.
- **Grade Group 2**: Gleason 7 (3+4).
- **Grade Group 3**: Gleason 7 (4+3).
- **Grade Group 4**: Gleason 8 (4+4, 3+5, or 5+3).
- **Grade Group 5**: Gleason 9–10 (4+5, 5+4, or 5+5).

The distinction between 3+4 and 4+3 is important because the first pattern (the "3" or "4") reflects the dominant growth pattern. Higher-grade cancers typically require more intensive treatment, often involving combinations of surgery, radiation, and hormone therapy. Lower-grade disease often allows for active surveillance with regular PSA testing, MRI, and occasional biopsies.

Understanding the Gleason system helps explain why two patients with "Gleason 7" may face very different treatment recommendations.

Overview of Cancer Treatment Approaches

Once a cancer is diagnosed and staged—and once its biological behavior is understood—treatment planning begins. Most cancers are managed using one or more of several core treatment modalities: surgery, radiation therapy, systemic treatments such as chemotherapy or hormone therapy, and, increasingly, targeted therapies, immunotherapy, and theranostics. The choice of treatment depends on the cancer's type and stage, its molecular features, the person's overall health, and the goals of care.

Some treatments aim for cure. Others aim to control or shrink the cancer, prevent recurrence, relieve symptoms, or maintain quality of life for as long as possible. Many cancers respond best to a combined approach, where treatments are sequenced or paired to maximize benefit.

The following sections summarize the major treatment categories, what they involve, and what to expect during each stage of care.

Surgery

Surgery remains one of the core treatments for cancer. It is used in several ways: to cure when the tumor is confined to one area, to remove lymph nodes for staging, to reduce tumor bulk when complete removal is not possible, and to ease symptoms or complications such as obstruction or bleeding. Modern techniques often combine diagnostic and therapeutic steps in the same procedure.

Before surgery, attention turns to **prehabilitation**—preparing the body to withstand surgical stress. An appropriate program usually includes exercise, breathing practice, nutrition optimization, smoking cessation if relevant, and strategies to maintain or improve sleep. These steps improve resilience and reduce complications. Surgeons also plan how to prevent blood clots, manage pain, support early mobility, and reduce risks of chest infections or constipation.

On the day of surgery, the anesthetist and nursing team review the plan and confirm consent. Modern pain control often uses a combination of local anesthetic blocks, non-opioid medications, and short-acting agents to minimize grogginess and support early postoperative exercise. Many operations are performed using minimally invasive (laparoscopic or robotic) techniques, which can shorten hospital stays and reduce postoperative discomfort. Some people return home the same day; others may remain in hospital for a few nights depending on the complexity of the procedure and their overall health.

Tumors are removed with a margin of normal tissue around them to reduce the risk of leaving microscopic disease behind. When lymph nodes are relevant to staging, a sentinel node biopsy or targeted node dissection may be performed. Pathology results—margin status, lymph-node involvement, and any biological features—help determine whether additional treatments such as radiotherapy or systemic therapy are recommended.

After surgery, the early goals are straightforward but important: getting out of bed safely, taking short walks if possible, maintaining lung expansion with deep-breathing exercises, controlling pain adequately, resuming eating and drinking gradually, and monitoring bowel function. Long-term effects vary by procedure. Pelvic surgeries may affect bowel, bladder, or sexual function. Removal of lymph nodes, especially in the axilla or groin, may increase lymphedema risk. Nerve irritation may lead to temporary numbness or tingling. Early referral to physiotherapy, pelvic health specialists, or lymphedema services often reduces long-term impact.

If a stoma (colostomy or ileostomy) is needed, either temporarily or permanently, dedicated stomal therapy nurses provide education and support. Modern appliances are discreet and allow most people to return to all aspects of daily life, including exercise, travel, and swimming.

Radiation Therapy

Radiation therapy uses targeted energy beams to damage the DNA of cancer cells, preventing them from dividing. Nearby normal tissues receive lower doses, and most can repair themselves. Radiation may be used alone, combined with chemotherapy or hormone therapy, or given after surgery to reduce the risk of recurrence.

Treatment begins with a planning appointment called **simulation**. During this session, imaging (usually CT, sometimes MRI) maps the anatomy, defines the target, and identifies organs at risk. Positioning devices or small skin marks are used to ensure each session aligns precisely. For left-sided breast cancer, breath-hold techniques increase the distance between the heart and the radiation field to minimize exposure.

Daily treatments are brief. The machine may rotate around the body, but the patient does not feel the radiation itself. Most people can drive themselves to sessions and continue many normal activities. Courses range from a few sessions using stereotactic methods to several weeks when treating larger areas.

Radiation can cause fatigue, which often builds gradually and improves within weeks of finishing treatment. Skin in the treatment area may become pink, warm, or dry, similar to sunburn. For head and neck treatments, the mouth and throat may become sore due to mucosal sensitivity. Pelvic radiation can temporarily affect bowel or bladder function. A small proportion of people receiving chest radiation may develop a self-limited inflammation of the lungs (pneumonitis) weeks to months later.

Brachytherapy

Brachytherapy delivers radiation from inside the body by placing a small radioactive source directly into or next to the tumor. Because the radiation is delivered at very close range, surrounding tissues receive much lower doses. This approach is used in several cancers, including prostate, cervix, endometrium and some head-and-neck or skin cancers.

Depending on the cancer type, brachytherapy may involve temporary placement of the radiation source during a short procedure (high-dose-rate brachytherapy) or leaving a low-dose-rate source in place permanently, as is sometimes done in prostate cancer ("seed" implants). Planning is precise, and placement is guided by ultrasound, CT, or MRI. Most people go home the same day, and the recovery period is usually brief.

Brachytherapy is often combined with external beam radiation and can allow higher doses to be delivered safely to the tumor while minimizing exposure to surrounding organs.

Ongoing care includes gentle skin hygiene, moisturizing, avoiding friction, and pacing activities. Any new cough, fever, severe diarrhea, or burning urine during or after treatment warrants medical review. Your radiation team provides specific instructions tailored to the area treated.

Chemotherapy

Chemotherapy uses medicines that circulate through the bloodstream to kill or slow rapidly dividing cells. These drugs are used in several settings: to cure, to prevent recurrence after surgery, to shrink a tumor before local treatment, or to control symptoms and prolong life when cure is not possible.

Chemotherapy is given in **cycles**, with rest periods that allow normal tissues to recover. It is typically administered through a cannula in the arm, a PICC line, or a port-a-cath placed under the skin. Before the first infusion, clinicians review current medications to avoid harmful interactions, discuss anti-nausea plans, and cover practical topics such as driving, work, fertility preservation, and vaccinations. Laboratory tests ensure blood counts and organ function are safe for treatment.

On infusion days, premedications are often given to prevent nausea or allergic reactions. Many regimens are delivered in day-treatment units; others may require overnight infusions. After treatment, self-care includes hand hygiene, avoiding sick contacts when blood counts are low, maintaining hydration, and recognizing symptoms that require urgent care.

Side effects vary. Fatigue is common. Nausea and vomiting can occur, though they are far better controlled than in the past due to modern antiemetics. Taste changes, mouth soreness, diarrhea or constipation, and temporary hair loss may occur depending on the regimen. Some drugs cause **peripheral neuropathy**, resulting in numbness or tingling in the hands or feet; dose adjustments may be needed to protect long-term function. "Chemo brain," characterized by slower thinking or concentration difficulty, is usually temporary. Scalp cooling may reduce hair loss for specific regimens, though it is not suitable for everyone.

Growth-factor injections can reduce the risk of severe neutropenia in high-risk regimens. Keeping a simple symptom diary helps the team adjust doses and support medications for future cycles.

Hormone (Endocrine) Therapy

Some cancers depend on hormones for growth. In breast cancer, medications such as tamoxifen or aromatase inhibitors block estrogen receptors or reduce estrogen production. In some premenopausal women, temporary ovarian suppression enhances treatment. In prostate cancer, androgen deprivation therapy (ADT) reduces testosterone to very low levels; additional agents may block the androgen receptor more completely.

Because these treatments alter hormone levels, side effects reflect a low-hormone state. Common effects include hot flushes, changes in sexual function, mood shifts, joint stiffness, weight gain, increases in visceral fat, and changes in cholesterol or blood sugar. Bone thinning is a recognized risk, making bone-health assessment (including DEXA scans), resistance training, impact loading, calcium and vitamin D when indicated, and lifestyle support essential components of care.

In some men with stable prostate cancer, intermittent ADT may be used to improve quality of life while maintaining disease control.

Lymphedema Awareness

Lymphedema can occur after lymph node surgery or radiotherapy. Early signs include swelling, heaviness, aching, or a feeling of tightness in the affected limb. Rings, watches, or clothing may feel tighter.

Effective management begins with awareness. Regular gentle exercise helps lymph flow. Good skin care prevents infections that can worsen swelling. If lymphedema develops, early referral to a trained lymphedema physiotherapist for compression therapy, massage, and exercise programs is important.

Targeted Therapy

Targeted therapies act on specific molecular pathways or vulnerabilities in cancer cells. Unlike traditional chemotherapy, which affects all rapidly dividing cells, targeted drugs interfere with particular proteins or signaling systems.

Tyrosine kinase inhibitors (TKIs) block growth pathways in cancers such as EGFR-mutated lung cancer or certain sarcomas. Anti-angiogenic agents cut off a tumor's blood supply. PARP inhibitors exploit defects in DNA repair, particularly in BRCA-related cancers. CDK4/6 inhibitors are increasingly used in hormone-receptor-positive breast cancer.

Side effects reflect the targeted pathways. Some drugs cause rashes or dry skin; others lead to diarrhea, mouth sores, elevated blood pressure, or changes in thyroid function. Monitoring allows early detection and management. Dose adjustments are common and help people stay on treatment longer with fewer complications. Adherence is especially important with oral targeted agents.

Immunotherapy

Immunotherapy enhances the ability of the immune system to recognize and attack cancer cells. Checkpoint inhibitors block proteins that normally act as brakes on T cells, such as PD-1, PD-L1, and CTLA-4. When effective, immunotherapy can produce deep and durable responses.

Because these drugs activate the immune system, they can cause inflammation in healthy organs. Immune-related side effects may involve the lungs, gut, liver, skin, thyroid, or other glands. Symptoms such as persistent diarrhea, cough, shortness of breath, jaundice, severe fatigue, headaches, or new rashes should be reported promptly. Early treatment, often with steroids, is critical and usually effective. Many people can restart therapy after recovery; others may achieve long-term disease control without further doses.

People receiving immunotherapy are often given a treatment information card to carry, so urgent-care teams know the type of therapy and potential complications.

Theranostics

Theranostics pairs a diagnostic scan with a targeted radioactive therapy. It follows a "see–select–treat–track" sequence.

First, a specialized PET scan identifies whether the cancer expresses a particular molecular target — for example, PSMA in many prostate cancers or somatostatin receptors in neuroendocrine tumors. If the scan shows strong uptake in the tumor and low uptake in normal tissues, a matched therapy can be used. This therapy delivers a short-range radioactive payload directly to those cells.

Treatment is given as a brief intravenous infusion in a nuclear medicine suite. Most people go home the same day. Precautions for the first few days are straightforward: stay well hydrated, flush the toilet twice with the lid down, practice careful hand hygiene, use separate towels, and temporarily avoid prolonged close contact with young children. Blood counts are monitored because temporary dips can occur. Side effects are usually mild and may include fatigue, nausea, or dry mouth.

The same kind of PET scan is used afterwards to monitor response and guide decisions about further cycles.

Clinical Trials

Clinical trials test new treatments or new combinations of existing treatments. They are not a last resort but an essential part of improving cancer care. Trials have carefully defined eligibility criteria to protect participants and answer specific scientific questions. Participation may involve additional visits or tests depending on the study.

Trials can offer access to promising therapies or new approaches to standard treatments. The decision to join is always collaborative. Your clinical team will explain the potential benefits, risks, and commitments so you can decide if the trial aligns with your goals and circumstances.

Side Effects and Supportive Care

Most people treated for cancer experience fatigue at some stage. Weight changes, muscle loss, bone thinning, nerve symptoms, digestive changes, and disruptions in intimacy or fertility are also common. These effects are manageable, and many improve over time.

Evidence consistently shows that exercise, cognitive-behavioral therapy, and mindfulness-based programs reduce cancer-related fatigue during and after treatment. Exercise — particularly when it includes resistance training and aerobic activity — also helps counteract muscle loss, improve mood, and support metabolic health. When fatigue is unusually severe or persistent, clinicians evaluate for contributing factors such as anemia, thyroid dysfunction, sleep disorders, depression, or side effects of medications.

Supportive care is always an essential part of treatment. It addresses symptoms, protects function, and improves quality of life throughout the cancer journey.

Key Takeaways

Cancer diagnosis and treatment rely on a structured approach: confirm with tissue, map the disease with imaging, understand the tumor's biology, and use these findings to select the most suitable therapies. Modern treatments are more precise and often more effective — from surgery and radiation to immunotherapy and molecularly targeted medicines. Across all stages of care, exercise remains an important treatment in its own right, supporting strength, metabolic health, resilience, and overall wellbeing.

This appendix is a reference to return to whenever clarification is needed. Understanding the medical framework helps you navigate decisions with greater confidence and supports the integration of exercise medicine alongside your oncology care.

APPENDIX B

Health and Exercise Professionals in Cancer Care: Roles and Scope of Practice

Introduction

The safe and effective delivery of exercise medicine for individuals living with or beyond cancer depends on an interdisciplinary team of qualified professionals. Each member brings unique expertise, qualifications, and professional scope of practice. Understanding these distinctions ensures that patients receive the right care from the right practitioner at the right time, particularly when dealing with complex cases such as metastatic disease or treatment-related complications.

Now I have to acknowledge that these professions, their training and scope of practice varies **markedly** across different geographies and I base this predominantly on the Australian health care system. So to any medical, health or fitness professionals reading this, let's not make this a turf war. It is unlikely that there will ever be enough of us to sufficiently support all those millions of people with or surviving cancer – unfortunately. There is more than enough work to do so I suggest we collaborate and do our best to bring the best exercise oncology to as many people as possible.

1. Clinical Exercise Physiologists (AEP, CEP, CSEP-CEP)

Core Competencies

Clinical Exercise Physiologists (CEP) or Accredited Exercise Physiologists (AEP) are university-trained allied health professionals specializing in the design and delivery of exercise programs for the prevention and management of chronic diseases, including cancer, cardiovascular disease, metabolic disorders, and musculoskeletal conditions.

Scope of Practice

- Comprehensive health and functional assessments, including cardiovascular and musculoskeletal screening, exercise testing, and risk stratification.
- Prescription of individualized exercise interventions for people with acute, chronic, or complex medical conditions.
- Monitoring of physiological responses to exercise (e.g., heart rate, blood pressure, oxygen saturation).
- Collaboration with oncologists, physicians, and other allied health professionals in multidisciplinary teams.
- Behavioral counselling to promote long-term adherence to physical activity.

Relevance in Cancer Care

CEPs are the most qualified professionals to prescribe and monitor **exercise as medicine** for patients undergoing or recovering from cancer treatment. They are trained to manage side effects such as fatigue, sarcopenia, neuropathy, and bone fragility, and to adapt exercise according to disease progression, treatment toxicity, and comorbidities.

2. Physiotherapists (Physical Therapists)

Core Competencies

Physiotherapists (PTs) are university-qualified clinicians specializing in the restoration of physical function and management of pain, injury, and disability. They often serve as the bridge between acute rehabilitation and long-term exercise programming.

Scope of Practice

- Assessment and treatment of musculoskeletal, neurological, and cardiopulmonary impairments.
- Manual therapy, mobilization, and physical rehabilitation.
- Prescription of therapeutic exercise for recovery of strength, range of motion, and function.

- Post-surgical and post-radiation rehabilitation, including scar management and lymphedema care.
- Guidance on posture, gait, and mobility aids.

Relevance in Cancer Care

Physiotherapists play a crucial role in early and post-treatment rehabilitation, particularly after surgery, radiotherapy, or chemotherapy. They are often the first to initiate exercise post-operatively or after hospital discharge and are essential in managing specific complications such as **breast cancer–related lymphedema**, **pelvic floor dysfunction**, and **neuropathy**.

---

3. Accredited Exercise Physiologists and Physiotherapists in Oncology

Both professions overlap in the cancer context.

- **Physiotherapists** often manage **acute** impairments and rehabilitation in hospital or outpatient settings.
- **Clinical Exercise Physiologists** generally focus on **chronic disease management** including cancer and longer-term conditioning in community or clinical exercise clinics.
- The two professions are complementary and most effective when integrated in shared-care models.

4. Fitness Professionals

Core Competencies

Fitness professionals typically include **Personal Trainers**, **Group Fitness Instructors**, and **Gym Coaches** who are certified through vocational or industry-based programs. Their primary focus is to promote general fitness, strength, and wellbeing in apparently healthy individuals.

Scope of Practice

- Conducting general fitness appraisals and basic exercise instruction.
- Delivering group exercise classes and personal training sessions.
- Providing motivation, education, and supervision for healthy populations.
- Referring clients with medical conditions to appropriate allied health professionals.

Limitations of Scope

Fitness professionals are **not qualified to diagnose, treat, or manage** medical conditions, prescribe clinical exercise, or make therapeutic decisions for individuals with cancer or complex comorbidities.

Relevance in Cancer Care

When working under the guidance of a Clinical Exercise Physiologist or Physiotherapist, fitness professionals can support **exercise maintenance** in stable, low-risk cancer survivors. They can assist with community-based exercise, ensure adherence, and provide an ongoing social and motivational environment once the patient is medically cleared.

5. Personal Trainers (PTs)

Core Competencies

Personal trainers are skilled in exercise instruction, program delivery, and behavior change for healthy adults or those with low-risk health conditions.

Scope of Practice

- Delivery of structured resistance, aerobic, or flexibility training sessions.

- Basic health screening using standard pre-exercise questionnaires (e.g., PAR-Q).
- Progression and modification of exercise intensity for general fitness goals.
- Recognizing when to refer clients with symptoms or medical complications.

Relevance in Cancer Care

Personal trainers may form part of a broader supportive care network once patients are stable and have been clinically cleared for independent exercise. Collaboration with allied health professionals is essential to ensure exercise safety and relevance.

6. Occupational Therapists (OTs)

Core Competencies

Occupational Therapists focus on enabling participation in meaningful daily activities by addressing physical, cognitive, and psychosocial barriers.

Scope of Practice

- Functional assessment and energy conservation strategies.
- Prescription of adaptive equipment and environmental modifications.
- Rehabilitation of upper-limb and fine motor skills following surgery or radiotherapy.
- Fatigue management and return-to-work programs.

Relevance in Cancer Care

OTs are vital in improving independence and quality of life, particularly for patients with advanced disease or treatment-induced impairments. They complement exercise-based rehabilitation by focusing on **activity participation** and **self-efficacy**.

7. Oncology Nurses and Allied Health Practitioners

Scope of Practice

- Provide education on symptom management, treatment side effects, and self-care.
- Screen for fatigue, depression, and physical decline.
- Facilitate referral to exercise oncology services.

Relevance in Cancer Care

Nurses often serve as the **first point of contact** in identifying patients suitable for exercise referral. Their advocacy for physical activity as part of routine cancer care is critical for patient engagement.

8. Multidisciplinary Collaboration and Referral Pathways

Optimal exercise medicine delivery for cancer survivors requires a collaborative model:

Phase	Lead Professional	Support Team
Acute treatment / hospital	Physiotherapist, CEP, Nurse	Oncologist, OT
Subacute / early rehabilitation	Physiotherapist → CEP handover	Dietitian, Psychologist
Chronic management / survivorship	CEP (exercise clinic)	PTs, Fitness staff (under supervision)
Maintenance / community phase	Personal Trainer, Group Instructor	CEP oversight, peer support groups

Clear referral and communication pathways ensure continuity, safety, and progression from rehabilitation to lifelong physical activity.

Summary

Professional	Qualification Level	Primary Focus	Scope of Practice in Cancer Care
Clinical Exercise Physiologist (CEP/AEP)	University, postgraduate	Exercise medicine for chronic and complex disease	Design, deliver, and monitor therapeutic exercise for all stages of cancer
Physiotherapist	University, professional registration	Physical rehabilitation and function	Restore mobility, manage pain, post-surgical and post-treatment rehab
Occupational Therapist	University	Functional participation	Assist with daily living, fatigue, and adaptation
Personal Trainer / Fitness Instructor	Certificate / Diploma	General fitness and motivation	Exercise delivery for low-risk clients under professional supervision
Oncology Nurse	Registered Nurse	Supportive care	Screening, education, and referral

Final Perspective

The delivery of exercise medicine in oncology requires clear delineation of professional boundaries combined with seamless collaboration. Clinical exercise physiologists and physiotherapists lead the therapeutic exercise prescription, while fitness professionals and personal trainers provide an important bridge to long-term participation in the community. Together, this multidisciplinary framework ensures that every patient with cancer — from diagnosis to advanced disease — has access to safe, effective, and empowering exercise-based care.

APPENDIX C

Exercise Safety Checklist — When to Stop Exercise

I strongly recommend that you wear a smart watch with falls detection and emergency call functionality as well as keeping your phone within easy reach.

Learn and practice how to initiate the emergency call procedure on your smart watch and phone.

Whenever possible, try to exercise with others, or at least have someone else in your home or with you when you exercise.

This checklist helps you exercise safely. If you experience any of the following symptoms, stop exercising immediately and inform your clinical exercise physiologist, nurse, or doctor.

Heart or Breathing Symptoms

- ☐ Chest pain, tightness, or pressure
- ☐ Unusual shortness of breath or difficulty breathing
- ☐ Feeling dizzy, faint, or light-headed
- ☐ Heart pounding, racing, or irregular heartbeat
- ☐ Lips or fingertips turning blue or very pale

Muscle, Joint, or Bone Symptoms

- ☐ Sudden sharp or severe pain
- ☐ New or worsening bone pain
- ☐ Pain, swelling, or redness around joints
- ☐ Weakness, numbness, or loss of balance

General Warning Signs

- ☐ Feeling unusually tired or exhausted

- ☐ Feeling sick, nauseated, or about to vomit
- ☐ Feeling cold, clammy, or sweating excessively
- ☐ Headache, blurred vision, or confusion

Cancer- or Treatment-Related Signs

- ☐ Fever, chills, or signs of infection (temperature > 38 °C)
- ☐ New or increased swelling in arms or legs (possible lymphedema)
- ☐ Unusual bleeding or bruising
- ☐ Pain near areas of known bone metastases

If Any of These Occur

1. Stop immediately.
2. Sit or lie down safely.
3. Tell your exercise professional, nurse, or doctor right away.
4. Do not restart exercise until cleared by your clinician.

This checklist is provided for your safety. Please read carefully and ensure you take notice and act if you experience any of these symptoms.

APPENDIX D

Rating of Perceived Exertion (RPE)

Rating of Perceived Exertion

10	Maximal exertion (can't continue)
9	Nearly maximal
8	Very, very hard
7	Very hard
6	Hard
5	Somewhat hard
4	Moderate
3	Light
2	Very light
1	Very, very light
0	Nothing at all

APPENDIX E

Using Music and Video to Support Exercise

Exercise is easier and more enjoyable when paired with music or video. The right playlist can set rhythm and mood. Guided videos can provide structure and coaching. Movies or television series can make time pass faster on a treadmill or bike. Many patients find that combining exercise with audio-visual input reduces perceived fatigue and helps them sustain sessions for longer.

There are two main ways to bring music and video into your exercise routine at home: **casting wirelessly from a smartphone** or **connecting directly with a cable (HDMI adaptor)**. Both can be used not only to display the exercise prescription or interval prompts on a large screen, but also simply to enjoy entertainment while you exercise.

Casting from a smartphone

Most modern televisions (Smart TVs) and streaming devices (Chromecast, Apple TV, Fire TV, Roku) allow you to "cast" or "mirror" content wirelessly from your smartphone. This lets you project exercise videos, online classes, or even your own personalized program onto the large screen. It also means you can play music playlists, or stream movies and television series while cycling or stepping, so the session feels less like a chore.

For Android phones (with Chromecast or cast-enabled TV)

1. Ensure your TV and phone are connected to the **same Wi-Fi network**.
2. Open the app you want (YouTube, Spotify, Netflix, etc.).

3. Look for the **cast icon** (a rectangle with a Wi-Fi signal in one corner).
4. Tap it and select your TV or Chromecast device.
5. Content will play on your TV; you can still control playback from your phone.

For iPhones (with Apple TV or AirPlay-enabled Smart TV)

1. Connect your iPhone and TV to the **same Wi-Fi network**.
2. Swipe down from the top-right of the screen to open **Control Center**.
3. Tap **Screen Mirroring**.
4. Select your Apple TV or AirPlay-enabled TV.
5. Your iPhone screen now appears on the TV; play music, videos, or exercise apps as desired.

Tips:

- Casting is easiest when Wi-Fi is stable; if signal is poor, use the HDMI method below.
- Line up your playlist, class, or episode before starting exercise so you don't need to adjust mid-session.

Connecting with an HDMI adaptor

Casting is convenient, but sometimes a direct cable is more reliable—especially in homes with weak Wi-Fi or older televisions.

What you need

- An **HDMI cable**.
- An adaptor for your phone:
    - iPhone/iPad: **Lightning to Digital AV Adaptor**.

  - Newer Apple/Android with USB-C: **USB-C to HDMI Adaptor**.
- Optional: charging cable plugged into the adaptor so the phone does not run flat during a session.

Steps

- Connect the adaptor to your phone.
- Plug one end of the HDMI cable into the adaptor and the other into the TV.
- Turn on the TV and select the correct HDMI input.
- Your phone screen will now display on the TV. Open your chosen exercise app, playlist, movie, or streaming service.

Benefits:

- A cabled connection is very stable—no buffering or Wi-Fi dropouts.
- Excellent for projecting interval timers or guided HIIT sessions so you can follow prompts easily on a large screen.
- Equally useful for simply streaming a film or television series to occupy you while walking, cycling, or rowing.

Wireless headphones

One of the simplest but most helpful accessories is a pair of wireless (Bluetooth) headphones. These remove the need for long trailing cords that can catch on handles or pedals. They also ensure you can hear instructions clearly over the background noise of treadmills, bikes, or rowers.

- **For exercise guidance**: headphones allow you to follow HIIT interval cues ("speed up for 30 seconds, recover for 90") or hear when to change a resistance exercise without needing to stare at a screen constantly.

- **For entertainment**: headphones ensure you hear the dialogue of a film or television show, or enjoy your music, without competing with the whir of equipment.
- **For safety**: adjust the volume so you remain aware of your surroundings, especially if exercising at home alone.

Most smartphones connect to wireless headphones easily via Bluetooth settings. Once paired, audio from any app—exercise videos, Netflix, Spotify—will play through them automatically.

Making it part of your routine

Think of audio-visual support not as a luxury but as part of the exercise prescription. Seeing your structured program on a large screen makes adherence easier. Hearing interval prompts through headphones ensures precision. At the same time, being able to immerse yourself in a favorite television series, film, or music playlist makes the experience more enjoyable and sustainable over the long term.

Patients often describe that a 30-minute treadmill walk feels like 10 minutes if they are absorbed in a program, and HIIT sessions feel less daunting when guided by music beats. These psychological benefits are as important as the physiological ones for maintaining consistency.

Safety considerations

- Choose content in advance to avoid distractions once you start moving.
- Keep HDMI cables tucked out of the way to prevent tripping.
- Set headphone volume to a comfortable level that still allows awareness of your body's signals—breathing, foot strike, fatigue.

In summary: projecting exercise content, music, or entertainment onto a large screen makes sessions engaging and sustainable. Wireless headphones enhance clarity and convenience, ensuring you can follow instructions or enjoy distraction without interference from equipment noise. Together, these tools transform the home environment into a personalized training space—one that supports adherence, precision, and enjoyment.

APPENDIX F
Exercise as a Natural Pain Reliever

Overview

Pain is one of the toughest and most draining parts of cancer and its treatment. But here's something amazing — exercise acts like your body's own pain medicine. When you move, your body releases a mix of natural chemicals and hormones that calm pain, lift mood, and help you feel more in control again.

This natural process is called *Exercise-Induced Analgesia*, which simply means pain relief caused by exercise. It works through several powerful systems in your brain, hormones, and immune system — all working together to make you feel better during and after exercise.

You might start your session feeling sore, stiff, or tired. Unless you are really, really in pain or fatigued, try to commence your exercise session. Begin gradually, and as your body moves, warms up, and metabolism rises, these built-in pain-relief systems start to kick in. Often, pain and fatigue ease within minutes, and you'll notice you move more freely, experience less pain, and even feel less nauseated. If your pain gets worse as you exercise, or you experience any of the symptoms detailed earlier, stop exercising immediately, and ask your health team for advice.

1. How Exercise Reduces Pain

1.1 Endorphins — Your Body's Natural Painkillers

When you exercise at a moderate to strong level, your brain releases endorphins, natural chemicals that act like morphine but without side effects. They switch off pain signals, boost mood, and can even create that wonderful "runner's high." This usually happens after about 20–30 minutes of steady activity such as brisk walking, cycling, or resistance training.

1.2 Endocannabinoids — The "Feel-Good" Molecules

Exercise also increases endocannabinoids — substances your body makes that are similar to those in medicinal cannabis. They calm nerves, reduce inflammation, and make you feel relaxed and positive. These benefits usually appear after about 20–40 minutes of moderate exercise aerobic and/or resistance training.

1.3 Serotonin, Dopamine, and Noradrenaline — The Mood Boosters

Exercise lifts levels of brain chemicals that improve mood and motivation — serotonin, dopamine, and noradrenaline. These help you feel happier and more focused while also blocking pain messages before they reach your brain. Most people start to notice a lift in mood, energy, and alertness within 10–20 minutes of beginning exercise and the strongest effects are usually felt after 20–30 minutes of moderate exercise aerobic and/or resistance training.

1.4 Fighting Inflammation

Regular exercise helps control the low-grade inflammation that often drives ongoing pain in cancer and other chronic illnesses. It lowers harmful inflammatory chemicals and raises helpful ones that protect your nerves and joints. Over time this can prevent pain from becoming long-term or widespread.

1.5 Testosterone — Helping Pain Control and Recovery

Exercise, especially strength training, gives a short-term rise in testosterone, a hormone that supports muscle repair, mood, and pain control in both men and women. Testosterone enhances the effect of endorphins and reduces inflammation, so you get a stronger, longer-lasting pain-relief response. For people with low testosterone (such as during certain cancer treatments), exercise can help restore balance and improve energy, mood, and comfort levels.

The most effective exercise to boost testosterone is high-effort resistance training using large muscle groups (like squats, deadlifts, and bench press) performed at moderate-to-heavy loads for 6–10 repetitions with short rest periods of about one minute.

1.6 Central Sensitization and Graded Exposure

Sometimes pain persists long after the original injury or inflammation has healed. This does not mean the damage remains—it means the **nervous system has become sensitized.** The brain and spinal cord start amplifying normal signals as if danger were still present. This process, called **central sensitization**, can make harmless movements or light touch feel painful. It is common after surgery, radiation, neuropathy, or long periods of guarding a painful area.

The encouraging reality is that sensitization is reversible. The same neuroplasticity that allowed the brain to "learn" pain can also unlearn it. The most effective tool for this is **graded exposure exercise**—a structured approach that teaches the nervous system that exercise is safe again.

How graded exposure works

1. **Start below the pain threshold.** Choose exercises you can perform comfortably, even if they feel stiff or mildly uncomfortable, but stop well before sharp pain.

2. **Progress gradually.** Increase range, resistance, or duration by small, predictable steps. Consistency matters more than intensity.

3. **Pair exercise with calm breathing and confidence.** When the body experiences successful, pain-free motion, the brain updates its "danger map."

4. **Expect temporary fluctuations.** Mild increases in soreness are normal and usually settle within 24–48 hours. Persistent flare-ups mean the step size was too large—simply scale back and continue.

5. **Integrate strength, balance, and relaxation training.** Together they rebuild trust in exercise and reduce the brain's protective overreaction.

Over time, this careful progression reduces the volume on the pain signal. People often find they can move further and with less fear. The brain learns that activity is safe, and muscles, joints, and mood all follow. This is why I tell patients: *motion is not your enemy—it's your teacher.*

2. How the Brain Helps Control Pain

Exercise activates key areas of the brain that turn down pain signals — like your body's own pain-control switchboard. These include deep centers that send calming signals down the spinal cord to block pain before you even notice it. It also helps you feel less anxious or fearful about pain, which makes a big difference in how strong it feels.

3. How to Exercise for Natural Pain Relief

Exercise Factor	Typical Range for Pain Relief	What It Does
Intensity	Moderate to moderately hard (40–70% of heart-rate reserve, or RPE 4–6	Triggers release of endorphins and endocannabinoids
Duration	20–30 minutes (can be continuous or in short bouts)	Keeps feel-good chemicals elevated
Type	Aerobic (walking, cycling, swimming) or resistance training	Stimulates multiple pain-relief systems
Frequency	3–5 sessions per week	Maintains benefits and hormone balance
Progression	Gradual — increase only when ready	Prevents fatigue or stress hormones from undoing benefits

3.1 For Best Testosterone Response

- Focus on large-muscle exercises such as squats, leg press, chest press, or rows.

- Use moderate-to-heavy loads (about 70–85% of your maximum, or RPE 6–8) for 6–10 reps.
- Keep sessions short — around 45–60 minutes — and rest 1 minute between sets.
- Train 3–4 days per week, alternating upper and lower body, with rest days between.
- Eat well (especially protein), sleep 7+ hours, and avoid long, very hard endurance sessions that can lower testosterone.

4. Practical Tips for People with Cancer

Exercise is not a luxury or optional add-on — it is a core part of your treatment, working like a powerful medicine within your body. The right "dose" of exercise helps reduce pain, fatigue, and inflammation, protects your muscles and bones, and restores confidence and quality of life.

Aim for a structured and progressive program that challenges your body safely but meaningfully. Combine aerobic exercise (such as brisk walking, cycling, or swimming) with resistance training (like weightlifting or bodyweight exercises) to stimulate the powerful hormonal, neural, and immune pathways that control pain and support recovery.

You don't need to "take it easy" — you need to train smart and precisely, guided by your symptoms and energy levels. Even during treatment, moderate to vigorous sessions are both safe and beneficial when prescribed correctly.

Work with a clinical exercise physiologist or physiotherapist experienced in cancer care to tailor your program to your treatment stage and fitness level. Your goal isn't just to move — it's to train your body as your own internal pharmacy, releasing natural pain relievers, mood enhancers, and healing signals every time you exercise.

5. The Big Picture

Exercise is more than just movement — it's a natural, side-effect-free pain medicine created by your own body. It combines the power of hormones, brain chemicals, and immune balance to reduce pain, calm the mind, and restore confidence. Regular, well-planned exercise can become your most reliable and empowering form of pain relief — part of your personal medicine plan for cancer and beyond.

APPENDIX G

A Resistance Training Program to Get You Started

Well... if you are reading this appendix then you are champing at the bit to get started. Exercise is exceptionally safe when performed in the appropriate setting, with the right equipment and supervision. However, if you have not already done so, please complete the **Self-Screening for Safe Exercise** and if you answer "yes" to any of the questions in the first section, seek appropriate advice and support before commencing or increasing your exercise program. Also, please review the appendix **Exercise Safety Checklist — When to Stop Exercise.**

Here is a resistance training program to get you started. This can be performed two times per week and up to three times. If you wish to resistance train more than three times per week then you need a *split program* which I discussed earlier in this book.

Start gradually and work up in both sets and resistance. Start with sets of lighter weight and higher repetitions and then gradually increase the resistance. If there is anything you don't understand read or re-read the chapters on exercise prescription and resistance training.

Session	Sets	Repetitions Per Set	Repetitions in Reserve
1 to 3	1	6	4
4 to 6	2	8	3
7 to 12	3	10	2
12 to 24	4	6-12	1-2

Exercise		Notes
Squat	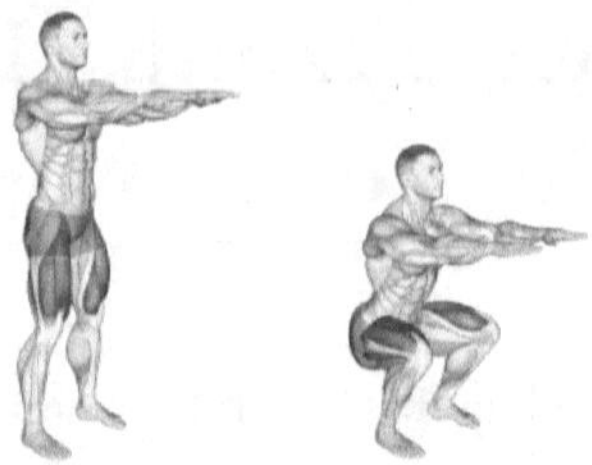	Just body weight to start with and add weighted bag or dumbbells held by your sides or at the chest.
Pushup	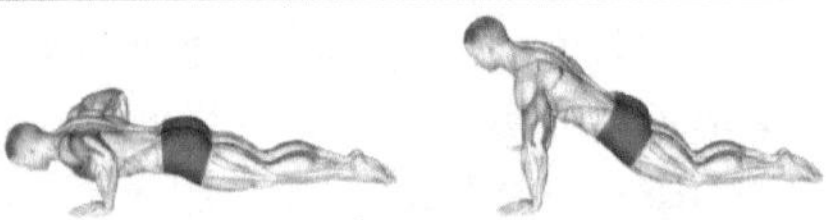	Perform from the knee position. Incline from a table or wall to regress or from toes to progress.
Deadlift	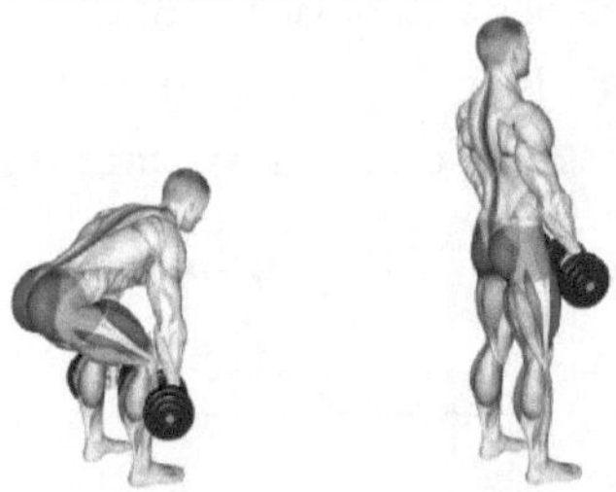	Start with just body weight and then add weighted bag, dumbbells or barbell.
Overhead Press	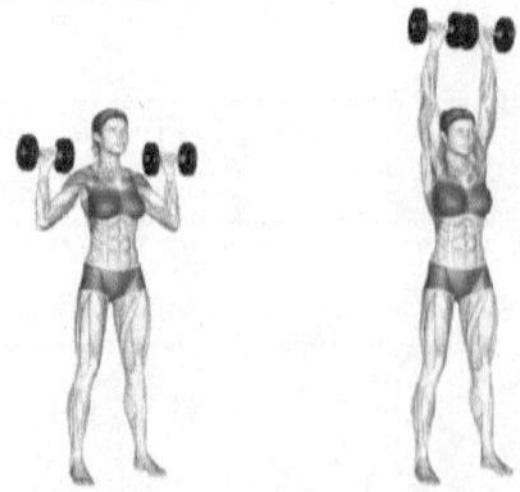	Use a dumbbell, weighted bag, or stretch band for resistance.

Step Up	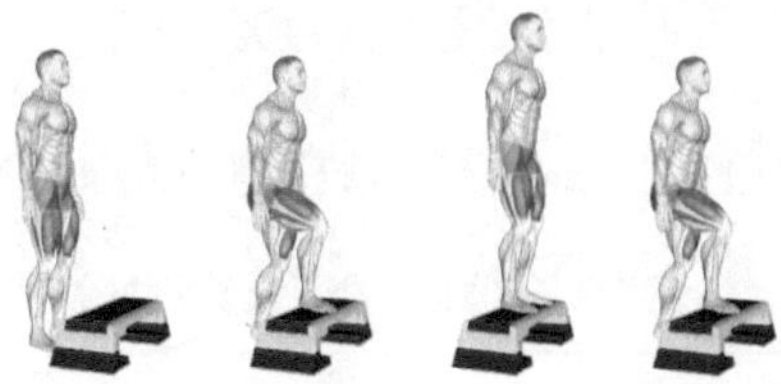	Step can be a bench, stair or any stable platform. Alternate legs or half reps on one leg then swap.
Bentover Row	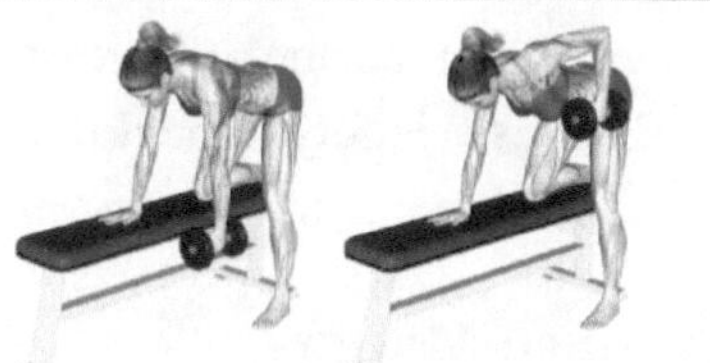	Use a dumbbell, weighted bag, or stretch band for resistance.
Calf Raise	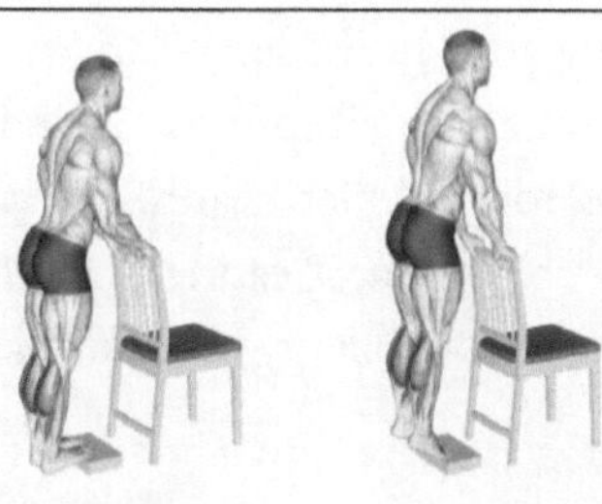	Elevate the toes to increase range of motion.
Gluteal Bridge	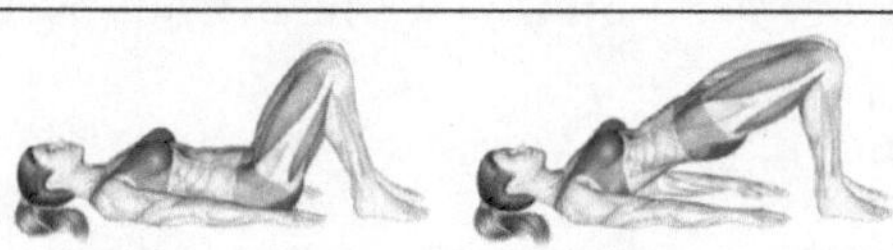	An easier option is to position the shoulders on the edge of a bed or lounge.
Forearm Plank	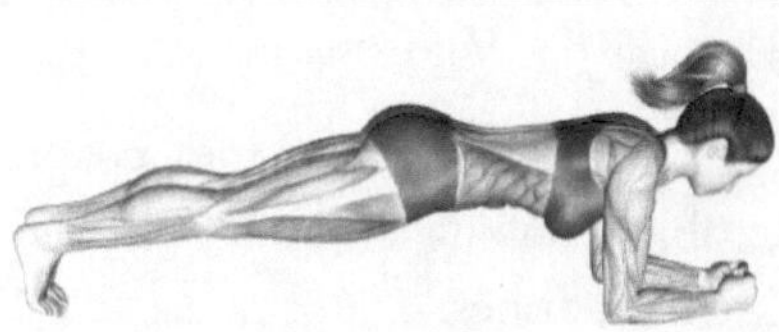	Hold this isometric position. To regress place hands on a table or wall to start.

APPENDIX H

An Aerobic Training Program to Get You Started

Before you begin this or any exercise program, please complete the Self-Screening for Safe Exercise form included in this book. If you answer "yes" to any of the questions in the first section, seek professional advice before commencing or increasing your training. Also review the section **Exercise Safety Checklist — When to Stop Exercise** to ensure you know when to pause or modify your session.

Why Aerobic Exercise Matters

Aerobic exercise (also called endurance or cardiovascular training) improves how efficiently your heart, lungs, and muscles use oxygen. It helps control fatigue, enhances sleep, mood, and mental clarity, and supports immune and cardiovascular health. For people undergoing or recovering from cancer treatment, it can lessen inflammation, improve treatment tolerance, and restore energy and confidence.

The goal is to start gently, progress gradually, and be consistent. Small, steady improvements bring powerful benefits over time.

Getting Started

Aim for at least three sessions per week, gradually building to four or five as you feel stronger. If possible, use a heart-rate monitor or smartwatch to stay within your safe but effective training zone. You can also use the RPE (Rating of Perceived Exertion) scale in this book: 2–3 = light, 4–6 = moderate, 7–8 = vigorous.

If anything feels unclear, review the chapters on Exercise Prescription and Aerobic Training especially for details on heart-rate reserve (HRR) and intensity zones.

Choosing Your Mode of Aerobic Exercise

- Walking — the simplest and safest choice, indoors, outdoors, or on a treadmill.
- Cycling — stationary or outdoor, excellent for low-impact conditioning.
- Stepping — ideal for home training:
    - Use a sturdy step 15–25 cm (6–10 inches) high.
    - A higher step or faster pace increases intensity.
    - You can use a commercial aerobic step or a household stair, ensuring it is stable and non-slip.

Choose whichever mode best fits your environment, balance, and comfort.

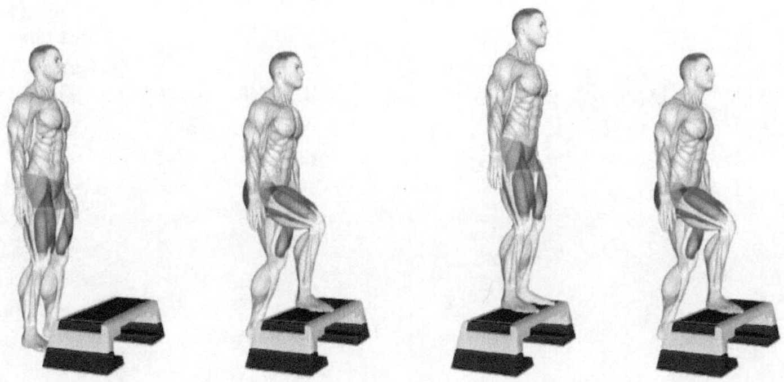

Sample Aerobic Training Program

Phase / Sessions	Format	Duration (minutes)	Target HR (% HRR)	RPE (0–10)	Notes and Progressions
1–6	MICT – Moderate-Intensity Continuous Training	20	30–39%	2–3	Begin gently. Focus on rhythm and posture. Walk or step at a pace that feels comfortable and sustainable. Progress by adding 2 min each week.

7–12	Alternate MICT and Interval Sessions (2 days MICT + 2 days Intervals)	25–30	MICT 40–59% / Intervals 50–69%	4–6 avg (6–7 work)	For intervals, alternate 2 min faster pace with 2 min slower recovery. Repeat 4–6 times. Adjust pace or step height as tolerated.
13–18	Alternate MICT and Intervals	30–35	MICT 45–60% / Intervals 55–70%	5–6 avg (6–8 work)	Increase intervals (up to 6–8 cycles) or extend MICT to 35 min. Focus on steady breathing and relaxed form.
19–24	Alternate MICT and Intervals	35–40	MICT 50–60% / Intervals 60–75%	5–7 avg (7–8 work)	Maintain consistency 4–5 days/week. On lower-energy days, choose a light MICT session or reduce interval number.

MICT = Moderate-Intensity Continuous Training | HRR = Heart Rate Reserve

Monitoring Intensity

Heart-Rate Method:

Target HR = Resting HR + (% HRR × [Max HR − Resting HR]) Example: Resting HR = 70 bpm, Max HR = 160 bpm → 50% HRR = 70 + 0.5 × (160 − 70) = 115 bpm.

RPE Method:

- 2–3 = Light (easy conversation and can sing)

- 4–6 = Moderate (conversation possible but effortful, cannot sing)
- 7–8 = Vigorous (speak in short phrases only)

Listen to your body — your perception of effort is often the best guide.

Warm-Up and Cool-Down

Each session should include:

- Warm-Up: 5 min slow walking or stepping to raise heart rate loosen joints, and warm muscles.
- Cool-Down: 5 min slower activity followed by gentle leg and shoulder stretches.
- Always reduce pace gradually to prevent dizziness or light-headedness.

Safety and Adaptation Tips

- Avoid training during fever, infection, or strong treatment side effects (nausea, dizziness, severe fatigue).
- Stop if you feel chest discomfort, breathlessness beyond normal exertion, or pain.
- On low-energy days, shorten or lighten the session instead of skipping entirely.
- Stay hydrated before and after exercise.
- Extend duration before raising intensity; consistency is the most important factor.

Summary

This progressive aerobic program provides a safe, adaptable path to rebuild cardiovascular fitness and endurance. Alternating moderate continuous and interval sessions balances safety with stimulation, supporting recovery, energy, and long-term health for people living with or beyond cancer.

APPENDIX I

Whole-Body Weighted Bag Workout

Weighted bags are a great way to resistance train that is low cost and can be done anywhere. You can buy a quality weighted bag online or at your local sports store. Choose one which is made of heavy, tear resistance material, with good handles and an assortment of smaller bags that you can fill with sand to create different weight ranges. If you need to be thrifty, then you can easily make a weighted resistance bag from a backpack and fill it with bags of sand. There are also bags that you can fill with water for resistance training.

Equipment: Weighted bag (5–30 kg depending on ability) Duration: ~35–40 minutes (including warm-up and cool-down) Frequency: 2–3 times per week, with at least one rest day between sessions

1. Warm-Up (5–8 minutes)

Purpose: Prepare muscles, joints, and circulation gradually increasing intensity.

- March on the spot or slow walk – 1 min
- Shoulder rolls and arm circles – 1 min
- Bodyweight sit-to-stand from a chair – 1 min
- Gentle side steps with arm swings – 1 min
- Light bag lifts from floor to chest (no press) – 1 min

2. Main Workout (25–30 minutes)

Perform one exercise after another as a circuit. Rest 30–60 seconds between exercises. Complete 2–3 circuits in total.

Exercise	Muscles Targeted	Reps	Notes / Technique +

			Progressions & Regressions
Front-Loaded Squat (or Chair Sit-to-Stand with Bag)	Thighs, glutes, trunk	8–12	Hold bag at chest. Sit hips back slowly, to squat to thighs parallel, stand tall. Progress: Lower deeper or increase load. Regress: Squat to chair for support or perform partial range.
Bent-Over Row	Back, shoulders, arms	8–10	Hinge slightly at hips, soft knees, pull bag to lower ribs. Progress: Pause 1 sec at top or increase weight. Regress: Perform seated, lighter bag.
Deadlift (Hip Hinge)	Hamstrings, glutes, lower back	8–12	Keep bag close, hinge from hips, then bend knees to lower the bag, stand tall squeezing glutes. Progress: Slow eccentric (3 sec down),

			increase weight. Regress: Raise bag on low step to reduce reach, lighter bag.
Overhead Press	Shoulders, arms, trunk	8–10	Press bag overhead, avoid arching back. Progress: Single-arm press, heavier bag. Regress: Seated press to eye level.
Glute Bridge (Bag Across Hips)	Glutes, hamstrings, lower back	10–12	Lie on back, feet flat, lift hips until straight line from knees to shoulders. Progress: Single-leg or heavier bag. Regress: Bodyweight only or reduced range.
Calf Raise (Holding Bag)	Calves, ankles, balance	10–15	Hold bag at chest, rise onto balls of feet, lower slowly. Progress: Single-leg or hold 2 sec at top. Regress:

			Use wall/chair for support.
Floor Press or Wall Push-Up on Bag	Chest, shoulders, triceps	8–10	Lie on back pressing bag upward. Progress: 3 sec lower or heavier bag. Regress: lighter load.

3. Trunk & Posture Focus (5 minutes)

- Seated Bag Hold: Sit tall, hold bag at chest, brace core – 3 × 20 sec.
- Standing Anti-Tilt Hold: Stand upright, hold bag on one side, resist leaning – 10 sec each side × 3.
- Wall Plank Hold: Forearms on wall, engage core – 3 × 20 sec.

4. Cool-Down (5 minutes)

- Slow walk or march – 1 min
- Shoulder and chest stretch – 1 min
- Hamstring stretch (seated or standing) – 30 sec each leg
- Calf stretch – 30 sec each side
- Deep diaphragmatic breathing – 1 min

Progression & Modifications (General Safety)

Beginners / During Treatment: Start with 1 circuit, lighter load (3–5 kg), longer rest.

Improving Strength: Add a second or third circuit, or increase reps by 1–2 per exercise.

Managing Fatigue: Split session into two shorter sessions (e.g. morning & afternoon).

Safety Notes: Breathe out during lifting, avoid breath-holding, stop if dizzy or short of breath.

Summary

This refined weighted bag routine targets major muscle groups safely and effectively, enhancing strength, balance, and function while protecting vulnerable joints and the spine. It is ideal for people undergoing or recovering from cancer treatment and can be scaled easily as confidence and capacity grow.

APPENDIX J
The Future of Exercise Oncology

Exercise oncology has advanced rapidly over the past two decades, but the next decade will bring changes that make personalized exercise a routine part of cancer care rather than an optional extra. Much of this progress will come from better integration of exercise into clinical pathways and smarter use of digital tools that help clinicians and patients work together.

In many centers, exercise is already introduced early, at the time of diagnosis or during treatment planning. This shift recognizes that exercise is not simply rehabilitation—it is an active treatment that helps people tolerate therapy, recover faster, and maintain independence. As oncology teams, surgeons, radiotherapists, psychologists, physiotherapists and dietitians work more closely with clinical exercise physiologists, care becomes more coordinated. Prescriptions can be adapted quickly when treatment plans change, when new symptoms appear, or when laboratory results suggest a need for caution.

Technology now supports this integration. Wearable sensors and smartwatches can track heart rate, oxygen saturation, sleep, activity, and recovery patterns. These data give patients real-time feedback and allow clinicians to adjust exercise dosage remotely. Monitoring of vital signs is now 24/365 opening enormous advances in safety and fidelity of care. Tele-exercise sessions—guided by video or digital platforms—enable people in rural areas, those with low immunity, or those in palliative phases to receive safe, supervised exercise at home. For many, this reduces travel, increases consistency, and restores access when attending a clinic is difficult.

Artificial intelligence and predictive analytics are beginning to play a role as well. Algorithms can analyze patterns in symptoms, physiology, laboratory results, and activity data to estimate fatigue, anticipate recovery time, and suggest adjustments to exercise intensity. These tools will never replace clinical judgment or the patient–clinician relationship, but they will help personalize care more precisely and safely.

Advances in imaging and biomarker analysis are also shaping the future. Portable ultrasound, near-infrared spectroscopy, and simple motion-tracking tools can assess muscle quality, blood flow, and movement patterns. When combined with emerging biochemical markers—such as myokines, inflammatory proteins, or metabolic signatures—they offer new ways to understand how exercise interacts with cancer biology.

As these innovations mature, the goal remains clear: to make exercise a core, predictable part of cancer treatment—prescribed, monitored, and reviewed with the same care as any other therapy. The future lies in a connected care ecosystem where exercise prescriptions adapt to the person's biology, symptoms, and lived experience, and where digital support extends specialist care into every home.

Exercise oncology will continue to evolve, but its purpose will remain the same: to support people through treatment, restore function, preserve independence, and improve quality of life. Technology and clinical integration will strengthen these aims, ensuring that every person has access to precise, evidence-based exercise guidance, wherever they are, at all times, and whatever stage of cancer they face.

www.ingramcontent.com/pod-product-compliance
Lightning Source LLC
LaVergne TN
LVHW100251210926
848480LV00003B/894